FROM A STAGE III-IV CANCER TO RECOVERY

FROM A STAGE III-IV CANCER TO RECOVERY
TESTIMONY OF LORD'S GRACE

Ambayeba Muimba-Kankolongo

authorHOUSE®

AuthorHouse™
1663 Liberty Drive
Bloomington, IN 47403
www.authorhouse.com
Phone: 1 (800) 839-8640

Published by AuthorHouse 03/04/2015

ISBN: 978-1-4969-6878-4 (sc)
ISBN: 978-1-4969-6877-7 (e)

Print information available on the last page.

Any people depicted in stock imagery provided by Thinkstock are models,
and such images are being used for illustrative purposes only.
Certain stock imagery © Thinkstock.

This book is printed on acid-free paper.

Because of the dynamic nature of the Internet, any web addresses or links contained
in this book may have changed since publication and may no longer be valid. The views
expressed in this work are solely those of the author and do not necessarily reflect the
views of the publisher, and the publisher hereby disclaims any responsibility for them.

Scripture quotations marked NIV are taken from the Holy Bible, New
International Version®. NIV®. Copyright © 1973, 1978, 1984 by International
Bible Society. Used by permission of Zondervan. All rights reserved. [Biblica]

*To my wonderful spouse, Ngabwa-Kabeya,
without whose endeavor prayers, commitments to
my medical visits and treatments and continuous
unwavering support in the hospital and at
home my healing would have been impossible*

*You were always by my side despite
your work load; May Our Heavenly
Father Bless You abundantly*

ACKNOWLEDGEMENTS

*F*irst of all, I would like to thank my LORD Jesus Christ for healing me. Sincere thanks are due to several medical doctors including specialized physicians, radiologists, resident doctors, and laboratory technicians, nurses and administrative officers, at the Ottawa Hospital, who worked tirelessly with higher level of professionalism and commitment for the recovery of my health. In particular, I am thankful to Dr. Oscar O. Simooya in Kitwe, Zambia; Drs. Claude Mwamba Mulumba and Lubumbu Kasereka in Lubumbashi, DR Congo; and Drs. Wayne Kendal, Rakesh Goel, Rebecca C. Auer, Joseph Mamaza and C. Murash in Ottawa, Canada for their endless diligent dedication to my health. They worked days and nights, weeks and months to years to ensure I recover my normal life. The commitment by our family doctor, Imani Bidari in Orleans, to my health has greatly been paramount in the journey for control of this cancer. The Ministry of Health of the Canadian Government provided financial assistance for my medical attention without which all laboratory analyses, treatments and cost of hospitalization would have been impossible. My sincere gratitude goes to many friends throughout the world for their moral, spiritual and financial supports. Considerable appreciations are also extended to nurses from Carefor and Bayshore Health Care Services through the Community Care Access Center (CCAC) for a well-focussed follow up home care that ensured my comfort and safety after repeated hospitalizations. Many men and women of God and in particular the ladies at the El-Rapha Women Ministries constantly pleaded to God for my healing throughout the journey of my sickness. I am heartily grateful to them. The support I received from my family, both my spouse and children, and other close relatives here in Canada and abroad not only has been crucial during this hard time but brought back the sense of life again into me. Finally, I recognise with sincerely thanks those unknown British and Canadian Airways flight attendants who continuously checked on me during my trip when I was urgently evacuated from Zambia for medical attention in Canada as well as those individuals who pushed me in wheelchairs to process my transit visa at the London Heathrow airport terminal in UK and the entry visa at Ottawa international airport. To all I say "I am eternally grateful for your endeavor to save my life as I laid critically ill and powerlessly in airplanes in transit, in the hospitals and at home."

Table of Contents

PREFACE

I never imagine in my life I will suffer from cancer, often thinking this sickness was a common encounter in the western world. I began struggling with a persistent high blood pressure, acute abdominal pain followed by intermittent rectal bleeding, and blood and weight loss. After consulting one of the local health centers for nearly about four to five months, there was no evidence of the cause of my sickness. Praise the LORD for I am alive though I had initially lost hope. He made it possible that I could reach another clinic far away from my workplace, despite considerable body weakness, where the initial statement on the illness identity was given and then to Canada for its final diagnosis. Medical staff at the Ottawa hospital, where I had been in and out for nearly two and half years, worked tirelessly and diligently to save my life and always provided high quality care despite numerous difficulties including severe impact of chemo-radiation side effects, surgical wound infection, kidney failure and almost dying after a 9-hour surgery to remove the cancerous tumor. But above all, I surely knew from the bottom of my heart The LORD, Jesus Christ, is with me and that He will turn around this desperate situation into a joyful one. As written in PSALMS 130: 1 "Out of the depths, I cry to You, O Lord", I knew very well – since my faith was at high heights – that He will lift me from down depths of valleys to the tops of mountains. Continual prayers and support from my family, and relatives and friends throughout the world as well as several pastors from different congregations not only strengthened and comforted me throughout the harsh journey of medical procedures and treatments but also acted as a strong medication to cure the illness. I say "thank you so much indeed to all."

CHAPTER I
INTRODUCTION

Understanding the nature of the illness

> *It may happen that cells in our body rapidly divide without control causing overgrowth tissues which in an abnormal fashion may result in a destruction of normal and healthy surrounding tissues and cells. These overgrowth tissues are often referred to as cancerous cells.*

*P*raise be to the LORD for I have recovered my health after being diagnosed with a cancer four years ago. For several months now, I have gone through acute hardship and discomfort due to various surgeries and treatments such as radiation and chemotherapy having considerable side effects. I do not know where to begin to tell you the story of my commitment to and consistency with medical consultations, laboratory analyses and medications in this journey to health recovery. The best way for me was to write this book intended to create awareness and inform you about the sickness, my coping strategies and types of supports I had built for my care that could be useful to you just in case—"I say just in case"—something similar to what I experienced happens to you. I have thoroughly examined what occurred to me, reflected exactly on what I have achieved and shaped ideas to share with others about my healing based on the experience of what I have gone through. The idea to write this book was born that very day I was told "you have cancer" and was profoundly influenced by the premise that the majority of the population, particularly in rural areas of sub-Saharan Africa where I come from, do not know this illness as well as a great deal of emotional and physical distresses it can ensure. In the ensuing I focused my thinking, despite the stress, pain and anxiety, to embark on a very difficult task to exactly relate to you numerous events as they unfolded during hospitalization and administration of treatments. In this way and that is my belief, you could at least learn something out of them which might be of assistance when such unusual circumstance confronts your life.

In biology, biochemistry, physiology, breeding and genetic courses during my education and throughout my career, I have learnt that microorganisms' tissues are constituted of numerous cells that increase in number ensuring the body development. For this to happen, cells undergo reproduction by dividing in a manner that maintains a balance between tissues. During cell division, one single cell always grows and divides to yield two more identical cells. Biologically, this process may result either from sexual reproduction called meiosis or general cell reproduction during which body cells undergo development and replacement or repair, such as in adults or after injury, also known as mitosis. In the later phase, the produced cells have complete set of chromosomes and the cytoplasmic material of parent cells whereas during meiosis, number of chromosomes from the parent cell is reduced by half to have only 23 chromosomes at the end.

In contrast to these normal patterns, body cells may rapidly divide without control causing overgrowth tissues and in an abnormal fashion could result in a destruction of normal and healthy surrounding tissues and cells. They are often referred to as cancerous cells (National Cancer Institute, 2006; Canadian Cancer Society, 2010). During this abnormal division, cancerous cells grow beyond their normal locations, invade other surrounding tissues of the body and finally may also spread to other organs. The transformation from a normal cell into a tumorous cell involves various stages including a progression from a pre-cancerous lesion to a malignant tumor. These changes are known to be the result of the interaction between a person's genetic factors and other external agents such as physical factors (i.e. ultraviolet and ionizing radiation); chemical factors (i.e. asbestos, components of tobacco smoke, food contaminants like mycotoxins and water pollutants like arsenic, lead etc.) and biological agents following infection from certain viruses, bacteria or other parasites like fungi. Cancerous cells can spread to other parts of the body through different pathways including the blood and lymph systems.

It is recognized that cancer remains the leading cause of death worldwide, accounting for 7.6 million deaths—around 13% of all deaths—in 2008 and about 70% of all cancer deaths occurred in low- and middle-income countries and will continue rising to over 13.1 million by 2030 (WHO, 2013). According to the World Health Organization of the United Nations (WHO), Europe and the Americas have the highest incidence of all types of cancer combined for both sexes whereas countries in the Eastern Mediterranean region have the lowest rates (Fig. 1 reproduced with permission courtesy WHO at http://www.who.int/gho/ncd/ mortality morbidity/cancer text/en/index.html).

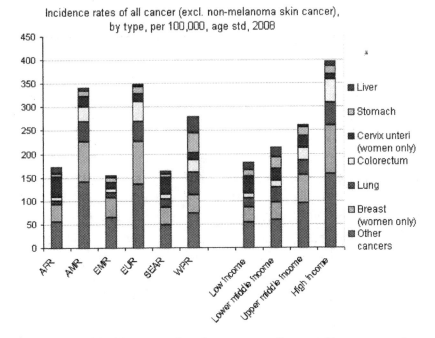

Incidence rates of all cancer (excl. non-melanoma skin cancer), by type, per 100,000, age std, 2008

Figure 1. Worldwide rates of various cancer diseases (Source: courtesy WHO, 2013. All Rights Reserved)

WHO states that women in its European Region had the highest rates of breast cancer followed by the Americas and all together these rates are more than double those of the other WHO regions. Men from the Americas Region had the highest rates of prostate cancer followed by those from European Region and the lowest rate of prostate cancer was found in South East Asia Region. The International Agency for Research on Cancer (2013) provided estimates showing that there were around the globe in 2012 about 14.1 million new cases of cancer, 8.2 million death that resulted from cancer and 32.6 million people who were diagnosed with the disease during the previous 5 years. Moreover, the Agency indicated that out of these, about 57% of new cases, 65% of cancer-related death and 48% of the 5-year prevalent cancer cases were in the less developed regions. From these data, there is no available information on cancer patterns in Africa, the continent where I come from. This could be attributed to several factors including lack of registries on the disease and necessary medical facilities for modern diagnosis and treatments in many countries (Parkin *et al.*, 2003). Moreover, they observed that there have been only few attempts to measure cancer incidence particularly among the rural populations, and when it has been tried, the recorded rates are low. In fact, many people die without seeking medical attention and therefore without knowing the real cause of death which may include cancer.

According to the National Cancer Institute (2014), "There are several types of cancer often defined according to the organs or cells in which they were initiated. The cancer that begins in the colon is known as colon cancer and that starts in the skin is called melanoma. However, these types are often grouped into broader categories such as:

- **Carcinoma:** A cancer that is initiated in the skin or in tissues lining or covering internal organs. It includes several subtypes, namely adenocarcinoma, basal cell carcinoma, squamous cell carcinoma, and transitional cell carcinoma.
- **Sarcoma:** A cancer that begins in bone, cartilage, fat, muscle, blood vessels, or other connective or supportive tissue.
- **Leukemia:** A cancer taking its root from the blood-forming tissue such as the bone marrow and causes large numbers of abnormal blood cells to be produced and enter the blood.
- **Lymphoma and myeloma:** Cancers starting in the immune system cells.
- **Central nervous system cancers:** These types derive from brain or spinal cord tissues."

Once they have been initiated, cancer cells have considerable potential to spread from the original site to other body parts where they can also grow into new tumors (Canadian Cancer Society, 2013). In this case, cancer cells that break away from primary cells are carried out to other parts of the body colonizing additional tissues and organs.

Many people are nowadays diagnosed with various cancer types, of which the most common are breast, skin, bladder, leukemia, lung, prostate, colorectal, cervical, childhood, thyroid, pancreatic and kidney cancers. Each of this cancer is important depending on the individual who is affected and may arise following numerous other factors such as the family history with cancer, poor diet, drugs, abusive intake of alcohol and use of tobacco, sexual activities, overweight and lack of exercise, and age with older people being more vulnerable. These factors also known as risk factors often act either alone or with one another, and some people than others may be more prone to any of the risk factor. Apparently, it has been found that cancer rates for all cancers combined are higher with increasing levels of country income. High income countries have more than double the rate of all cancers combined of low income countries and men have considerably higher rates of all types of cancer combined than women with the exception of low income countries (WHO, 2013).

Major signs of the sickness

Some of the early signs of cancer include lumps, sores that fail to heal, abnormal bleeding, persistent indigestion, and chronic hoarseness (WHO at http://www.who.int/cancer/detection/en/). Generally however, the following common symptoms can be observed when someone has cancer, but often they may differ in each patient and according to the cancer type. They are:

1) Weight loss for no reason;
2) Loss of appetite and severe discomfort during eating;
3) Constant coughing;
4) Weakness and feeling very tired; and
5) Breathlessness.

CHAPTER II

DETERIORATION OF MY HEALTH

Who am I?

Ambayeba Muimba-Kankolongo is a Congolese national born in Likasi, Katanga Province in the Southeastern Democratic Republic of Congo. I am the second child in a family of nine children. The first born, a lady, passed away shortly after the delivery of her first baby who

Suddenly, my health started deteriorating and I became very weak. Of concern were the abrupt loss of weight, anal bleeding and the rising of my blood pressure reaching at times 250-300.

survived and the third, also a lady, could not make it after a long hernia sickness. Both my father and my mother have also passed away resulting of me being now considered the head of the family. I am married to a wonderful wife, Ngabwa-Kabeya, nearly 30 years ago and together we have 5 children, the first being a lady and the remaining four being boys (Fig. 2). I hold a PhD degree with major in Plant Pathology and minors in Plant Breeding and International Agriculture from Cornell University in Ithaca, New York State in the United States.

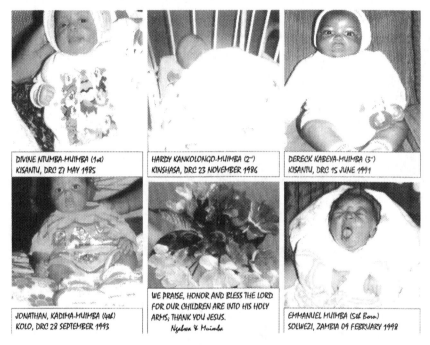

DIVINE NTUMBA-MUIMBA (1st)
KISANTU, DRC 27 MAY 1985

HARDY KANKOLONGO-MUIMBA (2nd)
KINSHASA, DRC 23 NOVEMBER 1986

DERECK KABEYA-MUIMBA (3rd)
KISANTU, DRC 15 JUNE 1991

JONATHAN, KADIMA-MUIMBA (4th)
KOLO, DRC 28 SEPTEMBER 1993

WE PRAISE, HONOR AND BLESS THE LORD
FOR OUR CHILDREN ARE INTO HIS HOLY
ARMS; THANK YOU JESUS.
Ngabwa & Muimba

EMMANUEL MUIMBA (5th Born)
SOLWEZI, ZAMBIA 04 FEBRUARY 1998

Figure 2. Our children when they were still babies

My graduate studies in the Department of Plant Pathology at Cornell have extensively enriched me both academically and personally, and have provided me with numerous benefits. I will say, concerning my personal perspectives on the value of education and instruction, that the Department I attended to in US offers graduate students a huge range of professional-oriented programs including a broader choice of well-selected courses. Faculty and associate staff are all experts in their respective fields of specialty and, more importantly, are all also very approachable and friendly. I really got the opportunity to enroll for many extra distinctive courses, never been offered in my home country, which were of great importance and wholly unique for sharpening my knowledge in the area of agricultural plant protection and for a well-rounded education that would better prepare me for the increasingly global world perspectives. Moreover, the updated nature of the literature resources available in both the departmental and main university libraries certainly facilitates the achievement of the student's education goals. Though I do not loudly claim to have become a sort of center of interest for efforts to produce more and healthy plants for agricultural development in sub-Saharan Africa where I have been working, I have recently observed my name being called upon for involvement in several international cooperative research activities throughout the continent.

I have worked for more than 30 years assisting smallholder farmers and National Agricultural Research Systems (NARS) in sub-Saharan Africa to improve food and nutrition security particularly for the poorest in rural areas. My career in the field of agriculture started, shortly after my Bachelor degree, as a researcher in Plant Pathology for a USAID-funded project "National Cassava Program (PRONAM)" of the Ministry of Agriculture in DR Congo in 1977 to 1992. From 1992-1994, I was nominated PRONAM Director by the Ministry of Agriculture and in 1994, I joined the International Institute for Tropical Agriculture (IITA) as Regional Scientist overseeing plant protection activities in another USAID- and IDRC-funded project, namely Southern Africa Root Crops Research Network (SARRNET) in Southern African Development Community (SADC) region. In 1998, I assumed the position of Director/Farm Manager for the Mukabentch Investment Farm Ltd. in Zambia up to 2003 when I was contracted as a Consultant by the Co-operative League of USA (CLUSA)-Zambia to train farmers' associations in Southern Province of that country. Starting 2004 to the November 2010 when I was urgently evacuated from

Zambia to Canada for medical attention, I served as a Senior Lecturer in the Department of Environment and Plant Science of the School of Natural Resources of the Copperbelt University (CBU) in Kitwe, Zambia. Zambia is a landlocked country, 752 km^2, situated in Southern Africa with the population of about 12 million. It is bordered by the DR Congo to the north and west, Tanzania to the northeast, Malawi to the east, Mozambique to the southeast, Zimbabwe to the south, Botswana and Namibia to the southwest and Angola to the west. My main interest for research has been crop improvement to develop high yielding genotypes which are disease- and pest-resistant for use by smallholder farmers focussing on rural household livelihood, and food and nutrition security and safety. I am author and co-authors of several scientific articles in peer-reviewed Journals, numerous papers at various conferences and workshops, and a book. I have considerably travelled to many countries in Central, Southern and Western Africa, in Asia, Europe and North and South America, and currently live with my family in Canada.

Beginning of the malaise

About four years ago, I started experiencing considerable health deterioration to the point of becoming very sick and weak. Of particular concerned was the continuous rise of my blood pressure, at times reaching 200-250, which prompted the medical physician at our local university clinics to request that I visit with him for a regular follow up on my health. Blood pressure is the force by which blood vessel walls are pressurized by the blood flow and it can have serious health effects. High blood pressure can damage small blood vessels as those in the brain, eyes, kidney, hands and feet. As time elapsed, I also developed a number of other symptoms including anemia, rapid weight loss (about 20-23 kg loss within a short period), vision changes, and sudden body weakness without enough energy including extreme tiredness and dizziness losing the balance when working. All these made it very difficult for me to perform my work efficiently. Following numerous visits and consultations with the physician at Copperbelt University clinic, I was prescribed drugs to take daily to lower the blood pressure. But this did not lower it; rather it was just rising to reach over 250-300 mmHg for the systolic target (the top number in the reading which is the pressure when the heart contrasts to push blood out) and 200 mmHg for the diastolic (the bottom number which is the pressure when the heart relaxes between beats) one day. This happened when my spouse was visiting me in Zambia. Because of fear of damage to the heart that could result from an eminent stroke or heart attack, I was kept under treatment at the clinic for several hours to lower the blood pressure.

Then, I observed poor food digestion leading to a severe abdominal pain and intermittent rectal bleeding often accompanied with mucus in the stool and internal anal itching. The doctor prescribed for me some medicines for hemorrhoids that I had to insert through the anus to minimize the annoying itching and pain in the anal canal as well as to end the bleeding during bowl movement. As days passed, my abdomen became swollen culminating in a prolonged loss of appetite. Any food including water was tasteless and it could not enter my mouth. My health was just becoming very poor prompting at one point the suspicion of being infected by HIV/AIDS mainly due to a considerable unexplained weight loss. I became so thin within a short period. Personally however, I was certain this was not the disease that has affected my body because of the negative result of the HIV/AIDS test I had just done few days earlier following the recommendation by the Canadian immigration for my permanent residence in Canada.

Because of the nature of our work both for research and lecturing, I travelled for a mission in the Copperbelt Province in Zambia and then to Lubumbashi in DR Congo for a research to study levels of heavy metals contamination of food crops by mining extraction and metallurgical industries. The research was commissioned with a grant from the British Government through its Program on Development Partnership in Higher Education (DeLPHE) involving CBU in Zambia and the School of Public Health of the Faculty of Medicine of the University of Lubumbashi in Katanga Province, DR Congo. Food insecurity in the region also results from the degradation of farming lands for agricultural production and the pollution of the environment resulting from mining extraction leading to food shortage and famine. Air pollution from mining tailings dust and emissions from smelter stacks all have had a negative impact on human and ecosystem health with by-products such as sulphur dioxide killing trees and negatively affecting growth of many plant species. Similarly, higher concentrations of heavy metals, such as Lead and Cadmium, have been recorded in various crops commonly used as foods in the area, often at levels exceeding WHO limits.

Unfortunately throughout the trip, I became unwell with considerable stomach pain, weakness and dizziness. The situation became worse particularly after the Kasumbalesa border post between Zambia and DR Congo towards Lubumbashi city. Seeing how I was struggling, my colleagues in the team advised that I urgently get medical attention at the University hospital in Lubumbashi when we arrive. As usual at the border between countries, everyone is supposed to have clearance with the immigration. First, we started with the Zambia side. We found a long line of travellers which made the situation worse because I was unable to stand for a long time on line. I was weak and feeling dizzy. I sat on the floor but was still uncomfortable. I tried to use the toilet but could not release the bowel. I was in general discomfort. Then one of my workmate asked for assistance from the immigration officer so that I could be attended to urgently because of my poor health. I was directed to another immigration desk where the officer checked my passport and the health card. I was rapidly cleared and then walked to the Congo side which was at about 3-5 minutes walking distance. When I reached there, I handed over my travelling documents to the officer in charge. He passed these to another immigration agent whom, I believe, was superior in grade to handle my case quickly. Surprisingly, I waited for about 15 minutes and no one called me for clearance. I waited again for about 5 minutes when I became impatient. Then, I asked

"Sir, what about my passport?" Without hesitation the officer replied "You need to pay $20 for your passport to be stamped for the transit entry." Because I was so weak and needed it urgently to continue with the trip, I did not ask why but just paid the amount requested. But, no receipt was issued. When everyone in the team received his passport back, we boarded the vehicle and started off. What was supposed to be a 1-hour trip becomes a very long for me as I was in intense pain. We reached Lubumbashi around 4h00 pm. I could not see the doctor that day since it was already very late for work. In the evening we went searching for a place we could have our super but I was unable to eat. I did not have appetite and I was in a very unbearable pain. I spent the night without closing my eyes because of the acute pain. Early in the morning the following day, my colleagues travelled to the various sites of the city to interview inhabitants and collect crop samples to be analyzed for our study. For me, I took a taxi for the University Hospital where I was among the several early patients at the door of the Medical Doctor at the clinics.

I was in severe pain during our trip and my workmates insisted that I urgently consult Medical Doctors at the University clinics in Lubumbashi town. I met with one of the doctors the following day who recommended for an echography test that revealed the presence of a huge mass in the colon.

Initial medical examinations

After consultation with the physician and physical examinations around the abdomen and in the pelvic area, he advised that I urgently undertake further laboratory tests including the echography and endoscopy. I went to the laboratory he directed me, but I found many people mostly women sitting outside waiting for the technician in charge for the laboratory. I sat down and waited as everyone. It took approximately 2 or 3 hours of waiting when one pregnant lady informed me that it is likely that this technician may not show up today. She said this was her second day of coming there without having the recommended tests performed. She then informed me that everyone here continue waiting because the tests are cheaper than at private clinics in town. If you can afford it, she said, you can go to the "Polyclinique le Jourdain" in the nearby vicinity where tests are done within a short time but at a higher cost. I consented with her suggestions and left.

I followed the direction to look for the address she had provided and found the location of this clinic easily since it was just few blocks near the University hospital. I introduced myself to the front desk and explained my needs. The nurse explained the procedure to follow and requested that I pay registration and laboratory test fees. After paying, I was given a receipt and told to sit and wait. I was called for the test after about one hour as there were many other people waiting before me. Unfortunately, only the echography test could be done there. After the test, the technician asked me to wait outside the examination room for the physician explanation. I was again called in the doctor office few minutes after. He looked at the echo image and asked me whether I experience anal bleeding after using the restroom. I said "yes." How is the nature of the bleeding? He asked. I tried to explain on my way. After documenting what I had to say, he instructed me to see the other clinic "Polyclinique Medical" just across the road for another endoscopy test.

When I arrived there I was asked to meet with the nurse assisting the physician I was looking for. After handing over to her the note from the previous clinic, she prescribed and requested that I purchase some laxatives to take prior to the test and to report at least three hours later after taking the tablets. I went to a nearby pharmacy to obtain the medication and went back to the hotel where I continued taking these pills accordingly. I returned to the medical center around 3h00 pm to meet with the physician. Surprisingly, he was not yet in his office and I had to wait for him for nearly another two hours when he arrived. I was called and he explained the procedure. Then, I was asked to undress and lie down on the bed with my face turned to the wall. A cystoscope was gently introduced in the anus for some times and then removed and re-introduced again to complete the test. He told me to dress up and return to the waiting room. Few minutes later, the nurse handed to me a sealed envelope with the findings and the recommendations to take to the physician at the university who initially requested the tests. I rushed back to the university clinic by taxi the same evening and fortunately found that the doctor was still in his office. I took a number and sat on a bench in the corridor where several other patients were waiting. About 1 hour or so, I was called in and handed over the envelope to him. He quietly read the report after he opened the sealed envelope. Then, he informed me that they have observed a rectal tumor (Fig. 3) of about 110 x 81 mm size that needs to be rapidly removed. He also indicated that I should immediately identify a qualified surgeon in Kinshasa, the capital city of the DR Congo, or in Zambia when I return back to this country to remove the tumor.

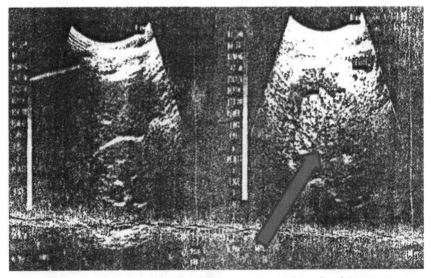

Figure 3. Images of the echography test in Lubumbashi, DR Congo, showing a large mass in my colon

I was shocked, frightened and suddenly began panicking I became so nervous and sad. I could not accept and believe on the results although they could not establish whether the tumor was indeed cancerous since the biopsy test was not performed. This was the darkest moment of my life I ever known. As devastated as I was, I returned to the hotel and informed my colleagues about the findings. I decided not wait for a minute to call my family in Canada and let them know that I was very sick and needed urgent medical attention as it has been recommended here. I did just this at the end of our mission in Lubumbashi. Upon arrival at home in Kitwe from Lubumbashi, I immediately called home in Canada and at the other end, my spouse immediately picked up the telephone. I explained everything including the recommendations that the tumor needed to be removed urgently. She then advised that I travel to Canada for further proper medical examinations to have a second opinion about the sickness. My daughter and she rapidly made flight arrangements with the British and Canadian Airways and transit hotel reservations in London as I had to spend a night over there and proceed to Canada the following day.

Before leaving Zambia, I needed to apply for medical leaves as required under employment regulations at the university where I was working. I filled in the leave forms which I returned to the office of human resources for estimation of number of days I am entitled to up to the time of my application. It came out that I was entitled to only 15 days having taken other days previously for resting. Since my objectives were to leave the country as earlier as possible for medical attention in Canada, I could not request for additional days at this time. I just decided to travel after my sick leave was approved.

CHAPTER III
FINAL DIAGNOSIS.

Travel to Canada via the UK

Flight attendants watched on me regularly during the trip from Lusaka in Zambia to London in UK. They were concerned about my health and were also wondering how and why I was allowed to enter the airplane. I was constantly praying throughout the trip until we arrived at the airport in UK very late in the evening.

I left Kitwe, where I have been working, at about 05h00 am on 21st April 2011 to Ndola by road and then to Lusaka by air, using the Proflight-Zambia Services, after I had secured from the Registrar Office, the previous day, some pocket money out of my accrued benefits to use during the flight and the first few days when I arrive to my destination. Within 45 minutes after leaving Ndola, I was at the Lusaka international airport ready to board the British Airways to UK at about 08h35 am. The boarding did not pose any difficulty as all my travelling documents were in order. I presented myself to the front desk and issued my ticket and the passport as required. After the airline officer took the documents, she pointed out that I did not have a transit visa to pass through London. After some discussions, she called one of her senior officers who indicated that I did not need a visa for UK. I felt released and went to the immigration desk where everything went well without problems.

We boarded the plane and after several hours in the air, I became unfortunately very weak prompting flight attendants to watch and monitor my situation more closely and regularly. They informed me they were concerned about my health and wondered how and why I was allowed to enter the airplane. I was constantly praying throughout the trip until we arrived at the airport in UK very late in the evening. According to my understanding, arrangements were that I will spend a night at Heathrow/Windsor Marriott hotel at the airport and proceed to Canada the following day. Since the hotel was at the airport I did not need to obtain a transit visa for UK. Because of the weakness, I was taken in a wheelchair to the information desk to ask about the Marriott hotel at the airport. Surprisingly, I was told the hotel was in town and not at the airport. I tried to argue but I was convinced this hotel was in town not far from the airport. Then, I asked the person pushing the wheelchair to take me to the immigration lobby to apply for a transit visa. When we reached there, he took all my travel documents to initiate negotiations for the visa focussing on my urgent need for the visa for medical treatments in the country I will be travelling to the following day. Fortunately and by grace of the Lord, I was granted a one-day temporary visa on humanitarian ground to get out of the airport. We went out of the airport and this person also assisted me in getting a taxi to go to the hotel. When I was there and with assistance from hotel officers, I was rapidly given a room near the front desk and the restaurant. However, I was unable to have my supper that evening because of severe pain. The following day, I was given a good breakfast in the room which I managed to eat.

Arrival in Canada

After the breakfast, I re-arranged and packed all my belongings in the room and requested one of the hotel waitresses for assistance to take my parcels where the hotel shuttle takes visitors to the airport. This was cheaper compared to the fare I paid for the taxi from the airport to the hotel the previous evening. Amazingly, I was able to walk outside to the bus place and to the immigration desk at the airport to process my travelling documents without assistance. Then suddenly while I was in the waiting lobby at the airport, the abdominal discomfort resumed with acute pain mainly because I was forcing not to go to the rest room any time I felt like bowl movement. I requested assistance for a wheelchair to reach the Air Canada aircraft to Ottawa. Shortly after boarding, something unpleasant and unmanageable suddenly affected my mood. I started sweating profusely and rapidly became depressed attracting the attention of one of the flight attendants. Two of them, a man and a lady, came quickly to my seat to establish what was wrong. I informed them about my health situation and that I was not feeling well. I explained the nature of the discomfort I was enduring. They gave me two tylenol pills and a glass of cold orange juice, but these could not help. From there on, they took care of me and constantly checked on my situation throughout the flight particularly that I had been brought in using a wheelchair. They regularly visited my seat to inquire on how I was feeling, served more water and juice to avoid dehydration and took me to the toilet where I tried unsuccessfully to release my stomach.

We arrived at Ottawa international airport late in the evening and I was again taken to the immigration lobby by wheelchair as I was now very weak, not able to stand or walk. I managed to submit my travelling documents to the immigration officer, a lady, for entry clearance. Then several questions were asked including why I was coming to Canada and how long I have been out of the country. The later question was asked because I had already my permanent residence a year ago when I visited the family for a short time. The rules are that from that time one should not spent more than 6 months outside. I tried to talk but my voice was faint and I barely open my eyes. She went through my passport to check for pages with the visa and the residence status, which she found. She then assisted in completing all the entry documents and the collection of my luggage. Thereafter, she escorted me to the exit lobby where I found my spouse. Realizing the condition in which I was; pale, incapacity to walk by myself or open eyes, talk clearly and particularly being on a wheelchair, she decided to call for an ambulance to take me immediately to the hospital. I requested that we go first home because I wanted to see the children. She asked whether I was sure of that. I said "yes." Panicking as she was; she drove faster home although I could not realize the actual speed and where we were passing through in the town. Within about 30 to 45 minutes we got home and all the kids were waiting. I hugged and kissed each one of them. They carried my bags inside while their mother was calling the ambulance. The only statement I recalled from my youngest son is "Dad you are so thin." I replied "yes, because I am very sick." I realized he was unaware of my illness thinking I just arrive to visit them as usual.

In Canada, my spouse has been praying day and night for almost 4 years since she arrived here asking God to bring the whole family together in the country. All the children had already joined her except I for sometimes. I remained behind in Zambia working as a lecturer in the university. However, few days before I arrived "she said", she spiritually saw that I started getting sick and that the situation was becoming worse. She did not know where to turn to but only to prayers because she had faith in the LORD's words knowing He is a Healer and also having a Women Ministries called El-Rapha meaning "God our Healer." This gave her again hope and enhanced her faith. Further, she looked in the Bible "she said" and found several other verses about healing and continued praying using those biblical words. [Psalm 107: 20] says that:

"He sent forth his word and healed them;
he rescued (delivered) them from the grave."

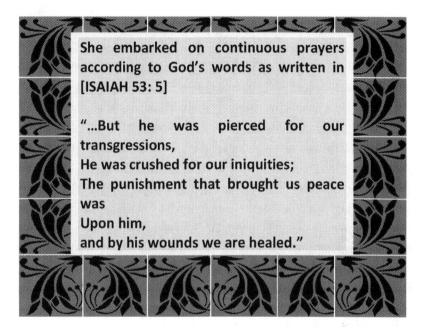

She embarked on continuous prayers according to God's words as written in [ISAIAH 53: 5]

"...But he was pierced for our transgressions,
He was crushed for our iniquities;
The punishment that brought us peace was
Upon him,
and by his wounds we are healed."

The ambulance arrived within about 5-10 minutes; paramedics embarked me in and drove up rapidly to the emergency department of the Ottawa General Hospital. During the trip, they were recording my vitals (i.e. heart beating and oxygen level, blood pressure, and the body temperature), constantly talking to me and communicating with the hospital on how I was responding. I was in really pain and discomfort. When we reached the place, I was taken to the front desk where nurses on duty rapidly recorded my complaints before I was given a temporary room in the same emergency department. Two medical doctors; one of them whom I recall was the radiation Oncologist, two resident medical doctors and a number of nurses arrived for physical examination, checking of my vital signs and collection of blood for laboratory analysis.

Medical examinations for final diagnosis

The Ottawa general hospital is centrally located in Ottawa and fully committed to providing patients with appropriate and consistent world-class health care including the best possible treatments for a wide variety of sicknesses. This is achieved through patients' care teams comprised of attending medical physicians, resident doctors and fellows, clinical managers, nurses, and several other health professionals such as therapists, dietitians, social workers, pharmacists and volunteers.

In the emergency department, my spouse and I provided all relevant information about my medical history and fully described the pain and discomfort I was feeling at that time. We also handed over the report of the results from medical tests at the University clinic in Lubumbashi, DR Congo which had indicated the presence of a mass in the colon. However, the biopsy of the mass had not been undertaken for the reasons that I cannot tell. A number of physical and radiological examinations and laboratory tests were rapidly performed including the radiogram, inspection around the neck and in the mouth, rectal and abdomen examinations, blood analysis for the level of hemoglobin and hematocrit, white and red blood count, mean corpuscular volume and hemoglobin, width of red blood cells, types of white blood cells such as neutrophils that are part of the innate immune system; immature granulocytes (small white blood cells containing proteins); lymphocytes that are important as they determine immunity types to any infection; monocytes which are destroyers of any invaders in one's body, eosinophils being responsible for combatting some kinds of parasites and basophils mediating the hypersensitivity reaction of the immune system; levels of sodium, potassium, chloride, carbon dioxide, anion gap, urea and creatinine, and others such as the carcinoembryonic antigen (CEA) from the blood sample that was collected.

The level of creatinine reflects whether or not your kidney is normally functioning. Specifically, the analysis looks at the body chemistry profile, markers of the renal function, cell counts, indices, platelets and automated absolute leukocyte counts. In the body, creatinine is produced from creatine, an important energy producer molecule. Creatinine is then transported through the bloodstream to the kidneys where it is filtered out and disposed of in the urine. In a healthy person with kidneys functioning normally, the blood creatinine is within a normal range. Hence, creatinine level in the blood is considered a good indicator of kidney function. When it is high or low, this could point out to kidney dysfunction or kidney failure. The CEA blood test uses a specific tumor protein marker associated with the colorectal cancer to establish whether someone has the cancer based on its level in the blood. The results of the analysis are compared with standards based on Hb S/alpha tha1 trait, which stands for the Alpha thalassemia trait. Alpha thalassemia is one of the world's most common single-gene disorders which range from the loss of one to about four alpha thalassemia genes in some affected persons (http://www.stjude.org/stjude/v/index. jsp?vgnextoid=d966885309c6f110VgnVCM1000001e0215acRCRD). Its syndromes have been found to be more common within African, Asian and Middle Eastern populations and are most prevalent in areas with endemic malaria. Based on the website above, different scenario as outlined below may indicate a person's health status considering the number of alpha thalassemia gene(s) he or she is missing:

1) One alpha thalassemia gene missing: this is a silent carrier which does not cause any symptoms.
2) When two alpha thalassemia genes are missing: This normally does not cause health problems, but can lead to low blood levels (anemia) and small number of red blood cells.
3) For people with three alpha thalassemia genes missing: This causes serious health problems which necessitate medical attention.
4) In case where four genes are missing: This constitutes a life threatening health issue.

Later during the day, at about 11h00 pm or so, the Oncologist doctor came in my provisional room and informed us that it is likely I am suffering from a colorectal cancer. Early morning the following day, a resident doctor, nurses and medical students visited to let me know that it has now been recommended that I remain in the hospital for a close observation, and for further medications and tests to ascertain the exact identity of the invasive tumor and the extent of its development within the colon. I was then transferred to a permanent inpatient room in the seventh floor from where I was subjected to numerous physical examinations and laboratory tests. These included chest and pelvis X-ray tests, a flexible sigmoidoscopy and colonoscopy, the computer tomography (CT) scan of the abdomen and the pelvis with or without intravenous contrast, MRI, the surgical of some tissues and their biopsy to analyse internal organs and tissues in the fringe of the tumor in addition to blood analysis.

The sigmoidoscopy test is performed to visualize the inside of the anus, rectum and the colon for any abnormal growths, bleeding or any other unhealthy conditions. Prior to the test, I was requested to take enema solution to empty the colon and during the test, I was inserted through the anus a flexible tube. Using a computer program, the radiologist observes for any abnormal conditions inside the colon. Just as for the sigmoidoscopy, I also had a colonoscopy test which also enables the examination of the inside of the large intestine or colon. For this test, I was instructed to clean my bowel as follow: I had to procure and take laxative drugs 4 Dulcolax tablets and 1 box of Pico Salax or Colyte; have my breakfast the day before the test and then remain only on clear fluid following this. The purpose of these laxative drugs is to ensure a proper clearance of the bowel prior to the test. Dulcolax stimulates the bowel muscles while also accumulating water in the intestines causing the stool to soften and pass through easily and rapidly. Pico-Salax is a strong purgative to empty the bowel of faecal matter and secretions. Thereafter, I had to absorb only small sips of water until 3 hours before the procedure. It was at about 2h00 pm the day before the procedure that I had to take the 4 Dulcolax tablets and then the first package of Pico-Salax at 5h00 pm. The second package was to be taken at 6h00 am on the day of the procedure and following this, I had to continue drinking enough clear fluid. During the procedure, I was inserted a flexible tube about the size of a finger having a minus camera and lighting at the tip. The insertion was through the anus and slowly advanced in the colon up to the rectum. Again, observations are made inside the colon using a computer program to detect if there is any abnormal development.

The CT scan consists of a computerized axial tomography test which shows images of internal organs and tissues in 3 dimensions to visualize whether the cancer has spread to bones or other organs whereas MRI, which stands for a magnetic resonance imaging, is identic to CT scan in that it also produces 3-dimensional, cross-sectional images of the body using magnetic forces and radio waves (Colorectal Cancer Association of Canada, www.colorectal-cancer.ca). During the CT scan procedure (Fig. 4), I was given two large glasses of oral contrast dyes to sip slowly for 45 minutes each before I was taken by a nurse for pre-assessment of my health history. The taste of the contrast is really very bad but it needs to be taken to obtain clear images.

I was then asked to lie down on my back on a table sliding into the scanner. Once I was on a good position, the technician and a nurse went out of the test room to a separate room with computers to explain how the procedure will be conducted and what I should do during the scanning such as staying still to avoid blurred images. After the explanation, the technician then activated the machine through a computer monitor. The machine X-ray beam began to rotate around my body also asking for a deep breathing in, holding momentary the breath and then breathing out as many times as the body scans are needed. Thereafter, I was intravenously injected with another contrast dye and the machine activated again. After repeated scans, the test was completed and was requested to leave the bed. However because I was feeling completely dizzy with slight burning of the body, I was required to sit still on the bed for few minutes before being taken back to my room.

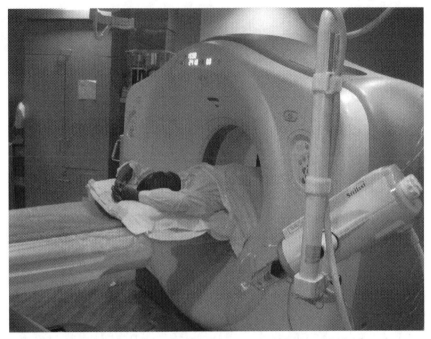

Figure 4. Lying on the back position on the sliding bed of a CT scan machine at Ottawa General Hospital in 2011

The biopsy was done by removing some tissues from the infected sites and examining these microscopically. This was the only way to determine with certainty the identity of the colorectal cancer I was diagnosed with and the possible extent of its colonization to several other surrounding cells or organs including the colon or rectal wall. From the findings, it was finally confirmed the tumor was a cancer in stage III to IV of development.

The MRI scan test uses radio waves from a circular magnet and a computer to generate images of the body area needed for the radiologist. I was asked not to eat at least two hours prior to the examination. In the morning on the day of the test, I was taken on a stretcher to the laboratory and once I was in the scanning room, the nurse assisted for me to lie on the machine table on which I had to stay still. The radiologist injected in my bloodstream the contrast gadolinium to increase the images' accuracy as well as a sedation medication which has the relaxation propriety. Thereafter, the radiologist, technician and the nurse left for another room to activate the machine through a computer. The machine bed was pushed into the circular magnet area while the X-ray beam was activated to spin around my body. During the procedure, the machine was also requesting for a deep breathe in that is hold momentary and then the breathing out as many times as the body scans are needed.

Several medical doctors including radiologists and resident doctors, and laboratory technicians and nurses participated to this effort. Nurses helped tremendously in lifting and moving me as my arms and feet were powerless to support my body balance when trying to stand. The final diagnosis from the CT scans and MRI images and the biopsy also gave indications of a stage 3 to 4 rectal cancer with a predominantly intraluminal mass having a rectosigmoid neoplasm of about 9.3 x 5.0 cm in longitudinal and transversal diameter. The mass was nearly causing a large bowel obstruction due to a significant proximal fecal loading (Fig. 5). Its bulk was more towards the right side. There were multiple enlarged lymph nodes around with the largest aortocaval lymph nodes measuring 15.0 x 8.0 mm, the largest paraaortic nodes 13.0 x 18.0 mm and the largest left common iliac node 14.0 x 15.0 mm.

Paraaortic nodes lie in front of the lumbar vertebral bodies near the aorta and serve for the reception of the drainage leaking in the region between the upper gastrointestinal tract and the other abdominal organs. There was a development of a mild to moderate right-sided hydronephrosis—the distention of the renal calyces and pelvis with urine as a result of obstruction of the outflow of urine distal to the renal pelvis and hydroureter—a dilation of the ureter—at the kidneys resulting from the mass effect due to the large rectosigmoid mass lesion. This large mass was also displacing the bladder anteriorly, but there was no evidence of its definite invasion.

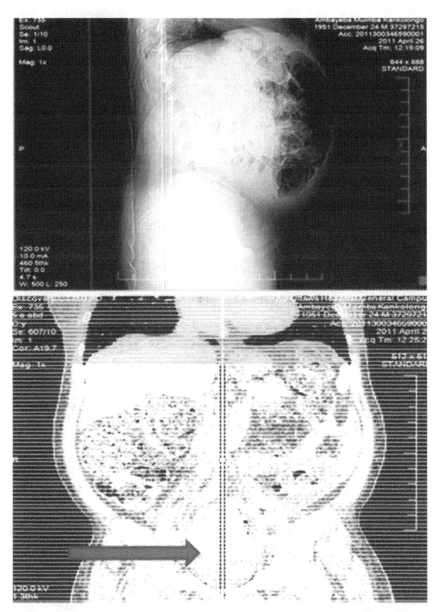

Figure 5. CT scan images of my swollen abdomen (top) and the cancerous tumor in my colon-rectal region (bottom)

The prostate size was still normal though there was some evidence suggesting the involvement of the right distal ureter secondary to the mass. Similarly, a large volume of air and fecal content were observed in the colon extending proximally from the sigmoid colon to the pouch at the beginning of the large intestine (cecum) and a relatively little fecal content in the rectum. However, there was no luminal air distension on the small intestine.

My lungs were well expanded with no pulmonary lesion that could be suspicious for any metastasis—the spread of the cancer from one organ or part to another non-adjacent organ or part. The size of my heart was normal whereas the thoracic aorta, that begins at the lower border of the fourth thoracic vertebra where it is continuous with the aortic arch and ends in front of the lower border of the twelfth thoracic vertebra at the aortic hiatus in the diaphragm where it becomes the abdominal aorta, was enlarged mainly as a result of my age. Moreover, several elements in the blood were not consistent with that of healthy individuals following various hematological investigations. From the above, I was put on category A for an emergency list to urgently receive blood transfusion. That afternoon, I was transfused a five unit's blood from the package mainly because of considerable low level of hemoglobin. The abdominal and pelvis scans revealed a normal liver with no hepatic nodules that could be instrumental to the development of cancerous cells. The bile ducts were not dilated and the pancreas shape was normal too.

More importantly, images from the MRI of the pelvis (Fig. 6) showed that the mass had already invaded several organs including the upper boundary of the rectum also known as the peritoneal reflection, possibly the seminal vesicles bilaterally, the pelvic sidewall with enhancement and stranding extending up to the right pelvic sidewall reaching up to the right long fusiform psoas muscle located on the side of the lumbar region of the vertebral column and brim of the lesser pelvis and the ureter. There was an apparent significant stranding and extramural tumor infiltration into the mesorectum with more than 5 lymph nodes that have suspicious morphology.

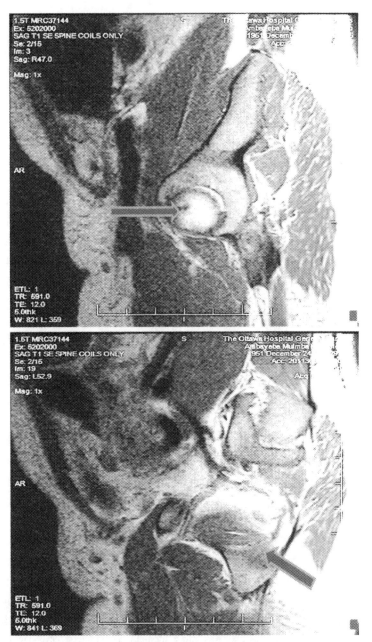

Figure 6. MRI images of the invasion of the upper part of the rectum (top) and some seminal organs (bottom) by the tumor

However, the left kidney and ureter were apparently not infiltrated. Physical examinations revealed other than for the abdominal distension with active bowel sounds and rushes, a no palpable swelling of lymph nodes around the head or neck known as cervical adenopathy. The chest was clear to the point of hearing any abnormal sound so was the heart. In addition, there were no abdominal guarding—the tensing of the abdominal wall muscles to guard inflamed organs within the abdomen from the pain of pressure upon them; rebound tendness—a pain upon removal of pressure rather than application of pressure to the abdomen; swelling of lymph nodes or inguinal adenopathy and lower body extremity swelling or extremity edema. I had continuous constipation with only liquid-like mucus coming out from the anus from a partial large bowel obstruction by the tumor causing acute pain on the right inguinal area. Unfortunately, bowel preparations for endoscopy tests were very poor to observe if anything of concern.

As the radiologist and nurses attempted to force and go further within the anal channel with the coloscope, a large quantity of watery fecal matter continuously spilled out the anus pampering the bed sheets. Nurses wiped me, collected the dirty items and provided for another clean gown. I was so sorry about the discharge while lying on the bed, but instantly all replied almost at the same time that it was normal since they face such thing from patients almost every day. Due to a poor bowel preparation, it was not possible to advance further beyond that point and no other obstructing mass could be seen to the hepatic flexure. The scope was pulled out. I personally believed this was as a result of fecal obstruction of the colon. In fact during the test when the scope was inserted in the anus, a profuse amount of faecal liquid came out continuously spoiling bed sheets and the gown I was wearing. It had a repugnant odor and was of blackish to greenish color mostly because I have been unable to evacuate any of the undigested foods for a long time. Regardless of the bad smell, nurses wiped it, cleaned my body and changed bed linens before being taken back to my room. During the process however, multiple biopsies were collected from the cancerous invasive rectosigmoidal mass for further pathological analysis. The radiation oncologist visited to my room very late in the night and said to us these encouraging words that keep coming in my mind and which I remember very well....

"Usually at this advanced stage when the tumor is likely already spreading over many other organs in the body, no one will accept a patient for further possible treatments. However, I take my responsibility to keep you in the hospital and try to do what best I could with other medical doctors to save your life." We said "Thank you."

The two oncologists, radiation and chemotherapy, at the hospital concluded that I will first need to have a bypass surgery before they could do anything. In this way, my intestinal continuity will be re-established to allow for the bowel diversion for feces and other waste to safely leave my body through an opening other than the blocked anus which is created on my abdomen. If I was potentially resectable by the surgeon from this cancer point of view during the above procedure, they hypothetically inquired, then they could administer me with infusional 5-FU or with IXO or also with FOLFOX plus A vastin chemotherapy regimen in addition to the radiation treatment for curative perspective to shrink the mass. They concluded that another surgery could be done thereafter to remove the tumor as well as several of the already enlarged diseased lymph nodes. However, in case the surgeon feels I am not resectable or curable from a surgical point of view, then they could only give me a systematic chemotherapy regiment. The idea was for them to be as much as aggressive as possible to save my life. Nevertheless, there was another major problem to the administration of the radiation treatment. The problem was related to the distension of my abdomen and the clinical signs of a continuing incomplete colonic obstruction I developed making it inappropriate for radiation therapy. If the treatment is given in such case, it could lead to a complete obstruct and also to the possible changing of the abdominal girth—the measurement of the distance around the abdomen at a specific point, usually at the level of the belly button (navel) which may assist mainly in diagnosing and monitoring the buildup of intestinal gas, most often caused by blockage or obstruction in the intestines—that could modify the whole treatment dosimetry—the measurement of the radiation dose received. To avoid this situation, the oncologists advised for the colorectal surgeon to perform the defunctioning colostomy by placing it away from the pelvis and out of radiation field. This was because the treatment would be coming up to the internal L4 region of the body where the tumor has already reached. At the end, they concluded that a thoroughly discussion by a team of multidisciplinary medical experts involving several doctors was needed to set up a comprehensive package concerning my medical intervention with well-defined tests, treatments and surgeries.

A constituted team of medical doctors was set and met to review my health and to statute on an aggressive plan of intervention. Following this meeting, the surgeon set a date for a defunctioning colostomy surgery at the Civic hospital for the end of May 2011 and the oncologists suggested that I should be administered a chemo-radiation regiment over a period of five weeks following the colostomy surgery after which I should be allowed for another six weeks break because of a huge effect of the treatments. Then following the break, I will undergo another surgery for resection of the rectal tumor if possible at this point according to how well everything will go. They hoped that lymph nodes in front of the L4 region would have been safely treated with radiation for them to be resected together with the primary tumor during the final surgery. I was called to meet with both oncologists and surgeons to discuss about the potential of a number of side effects and serious complications that might happen during and following the various interventions, particularly with respect to bowel complications which are experienced in 1 out of 5 patients considering the large field to be used during chemo-radiation therapy. Usual effects such as dehydration, fatigue, skin changes and generalized malaise as well as the possibility of the sacral plexopathy—damage of mainly the nerve plexus which provides the body motor and other sensory nerves for the posterior thigh, most of the lower leg, the entire foot, and part of the pelvis—was fully also discussed.

Development of colorectal cancer

Due to nature of the work I was doing, I could not initially think of something wrong had affected my health. Everything was going on well with my lecturing to students and my research activities in smallholder farms until, suddenly, I could not bear the burden of sitting long times preparing my notes and reports, and walking long distance in fields. As I had already indicated, I was regularly visiting the university clinic for my blood pressure that kept increasing to an alarming level not realizing this was not the problem but rather it came about due to another unknown issue in my body, at least at that time. The cancer that has affected my body, which is that of the colon and rectum or colorectal cancer, generally develops within one's large intestine (http://www.umm.edu/altmed/articles/colorectal-cancer-000026.htm). The human colon is composed of five different portions, namely the ascending, transverse, descending, sigmoidal colon and the rectum. Marks (2012) described the colon and rectum as the end portions of the tube extending from the mouth to the anus (Fig. 7 reproduced with permission courtesy AMA available at http://www.ama-assn.org//ama/pub/physician-resources/patient-education-materials/atlas-of-human-body/digestive-system.page).

When food is taken, as he says, it is first passed through the mouth where it is chewed and swallowed. Then, it travels through the esophagus into the stomach where it is ground into smaller particles. It then enters the small intestine in a carefully controlled manner where its final digestion and absorption of its nutritional contents take place to maintain the body healthy. The food that is not digested and absorbed enters the large intestine or the colon and finally the rectum to the anal canal or anus which is the opening of the large intestine to the outside of the body. Generally, any food that has passed through the colon constitutes the solid waste or stool that eventually finds its way out of the body through the anus. The large intestine is about two meters long and acts primarily as a storage facility for waste. According to the Colorectal Cancer Association of Canada (2010), nearly all nutrients from food are absorbed into the bloodstream along the length of the small intestine. They indicated that colorectal cancer begins to grow as non-cancerous tissues on the inner lining of the colon or rectum and slowly spreads within the colon after some times before becoming cancerous. Moreover, they observed that the cancer can stay in the colon or rectum for many months or years and if it is not detected and treated as early as possible, the disease can spread beyond the large intestine to several other parts of the body, first to the lymph nodes and then to other distant organs such as the liver, the abdomen or the lung.

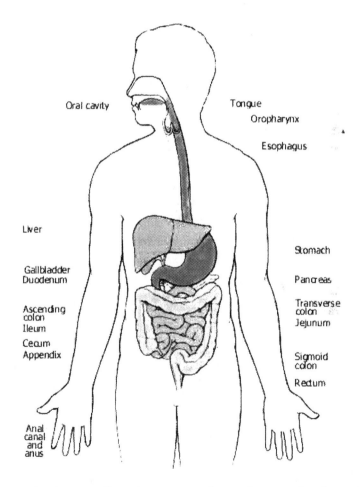

Figure 7. The human digestive system from the mouth where food is ingested to the anus where non-digested food is removed from the body (Source: Current Procedural Terminology, 1998 Edition, Copyright 1997 American Medical Association. All Rights Reserved)

In Canada in general, it has been estimated in 2014 that about 24,400 people will develop this disease and nearly 9,300 will die of it (Table 1, Canadian Cancer Society's Steering Committee on Cancer Statistics, 2014). It is considered as the second most common cause of cancer death for males and the third most common cause of cancer death among the females in the country. Based on current available incidence rates of the disease, the Canadian statistics office estimates that nearly 6.3% of women and 7.5% of men in the country will develop the illness during their lifetime and that about 11.5% of women and 12.8% of men, or approximately 1 in every 28 Canadians will die from colorectal cancer. The most common 10-year prevalent cancers among women are breast, colorectal, body uterus and lung cancers whereas for men prostate, colorectal, bladder and lung cancers are the most prevalent for the similar life time frame. The National Cancer Institute (2013) in US stated that spreading of colorectal cancer in one's body occurs via various channels including body tissue, the lymph system and blood.

Table 1. Person-based prevalence for selected cancers by prevalence duration and sex, and ten-year person-based prevalence proportions for the most common cancers by sex, Canada,* January 1, 2009

	Number of persons			% of Canadian population		
	Both	Males	Females	Both	Males	Females
All Cancers	810,045	406,065	403,980	2.4	2.4	2.4
Female Breast	158,405	1,045	157,360	-	-	0.9
Prostate	176,355	176,355	-	-	1.1	-
Colorectal	104,130	55,985	48,145	0.3	0.3	0.3
Lung*	39,115	18,335	20,775	0.1	0.1	0.1

- Not applicable; analysis by: Health Statistics Canada
* Prevalence estimates may be lower than in previous publication due to different method to estimate Quebec's prevalence prior to 2013
(Source: Adapted from Canadian Cancer Registry database at Statistics Canada, Canadian Cancer Society's Steering Committee on Cancer Statistics, 2014)

The disease undergoes developmental progression from its initial infection which is known as stages of cancer. These stages are well recognised following the examination of tissue samples by pathologists. They include the followings as described by the National Cancer Institute: PDQ® (2013).

Stage 0 or Carcinoma in Situ: In this stage, abnormal cells are found in the mucosa—moist tissue lining certain parts of one's body—of the colon wall and may become cancer and spread.

Stage I: Here, the cancer has formed in the mucosa innermost layer of the colon wall and has spread to the layer of tissues under the mucosa.

It may have also spread to the muscle layer of the colon wall.

Stage II: This stage is divided into stages IIA, IIB and IIC.

- **Stage IIA**: Cancer has spread through the muscle layer of the colon wall to the serosa, outermost layer, of the colon wall.
- **Stage IIB**: Cancer has spread through the serosa, outmost layer, of the colon wall but has not spread to nearby organs.
- **Stage IIC**: Cancer has spread through the serosa, outermost layer, of the colon wall to nearby organs.

Stage III: This stage is divided into stages IIIA, IIIB and IIIC.

A) **Stage IIIA**

- Cancer may have spread through the mucosa which is the innermost layer of the colon wall to the layer under the mucosa and may have spread to the muscle layer of the colon wall. It has also spread to at least one but not more than 3 nearby lymph nodes or cancer cells have formed in tissues near the lymph nodes; or

- Cancer has spread through the mucosa, innermost layer, of the colon wall to the layer of tissue under the mucosa;
- Cancer has spread to at least 4 but not more than 6 nearby lymph nodes.

B) Stage IIIB

- Cancer has spread through the muscle layer of the colon wall to the serosa of the colon wall or has spread through the serosa but not to nearby organs. It has spread to at least one but not more than 3 nearby lymph nodes or cancer cells have formed in tissues near the lymph nodes; or
- Cancer has spread to the muscle layer of the colon wall or to the serosa of the colon wall. It has spread to at least 4 but not more than 6 lymph nodes: or
- Cancer has spread through the mucosa of the colon wall to the layer of tissue under the mucosa and may have spread to the muscle layer of the colon wall. Cancer has spread to 7 or more nearby lymph nodes.

C) Stage IIIC

- Cancer has spread through the serosa of the colon wall but has not spread to nearby organs. It has spread to at least 4 but not more than 6 nearby lymph nodes; or
- Cancer has spread through the muscle layer of the colon wall to the serosa of the colon wall or has spread through the serosa but has not spread to nearby organs. I has spread to 7 or more nearby lymph nodes; or
- Cancer has spread through the serosa of the colon wall and has spread to nearby organs. It has spread to one or more nearby lymph nodes or cancer cells have formed in tissues near the lymph nodes.

Stage IV: It is divided into stages IVA and IVB.

A) **Stage IVA**

- Cancer may have spread through the colon wall and may have spread to nearby organs or lymph nodes. It has spread to one organ that is not near the colon, such as the liver, lung, or ovary, or to a distant lymph node.

B) **Stage IVB**

- Cancer may have spread through the colon wall and may have spread to nearby organs or lymph nodes. It has spread to more than one organ that is not near the colon or into the lining of the abdominal wall.

The higher the level of the tumor, the more advanced is someone's cancer and knowing the stage of disease development is necessary for establishing its best treatment protocols which may be one or a combination of two or more treatments."

CHAPTER IV

REVIEWING MY PAST

Causes of my sickness

T hough I was happy with such approach of treatments as proposed by the hospital, I felt however very much apart with my heart being greatly broken because of the diagnostic results. I

> *From my family side, I have lost my father and my mother, and two sisters, one before me and the other after me but all died from other health issues than cancer.*

constantly asked myself several questions that came to my mind. Some of these were:

"Is really this sickness in my family's

history tree?"

"Have I lost some family members from cancer who I do not recall?"

"What is my future going to be?"

"What is going to happen to my family?"

"Who will take care of the children and the spouse in case of my death?"

"Are the proposed treatments going to work on me?"

"How long these will take?"

"What about my work that I loved so much?"

"Should I return again to Africa if I am healed?"

"If not, when will I secure another job here in Canada to sustain my family?"

"Am I going to lose all my friends because of this sickness?"

"Should I tell them and my other relatives back in my country of origin in Africa about it?"

I was considerably emotionally distressed and I considered this as the darkest moment of my life I ever known. A week later I was discharged from the hospital to wait from home for the outcome of discussions by medical doctors about my next medical attention. However while with the oncologists, I enquired on the possible origin of the illness based on their expertise and due to their own encounters with several other cancer patients. They advanced a number of possible scenarios that could explain the development of this disease in my body, but they were not certain of the exact cause in my case. They explained that a cancer disease could derive from various ways. Some of the major causes of cancer that have been well documented include family history of the sickness, eating habits of certain types of unhealthy foods, abrupt genetic mutation in one's body and several others such as lack of physical exercises, smoking and alcoholism. From the explanations given, I started examining my past to identify where the illness might have originated.

I am born in a family of nine children and the second out of them. Among these, five are boys and four girls. My parents have all passed away due to their old age and to my knowledge, they never experienced a sickness one could characterize as cancer considering what I now know. My father has been a wonderful and loving person. He worked as a mechanics and despite his low income, he always made sure his household's needs – foods; clothing; educational assets at least at primary and secondary schools; medical attention that he could afford; and either a rental home in cities or a hut in the village – were met. After he retired from his mechanical employment in Likasi and Lubumbashi towns, south of the DR Congo in the Katanga Province, he moved with the whole family to our village "Bena Mbayi Tshipadi" in Miabi District, Eastern Kasaï Province. There, he engaged in farming as a new life to sustain the family up to his old age when he passed away. Unfortunately, I was unable to attend to his funeral due to civil unrest and war in Congo during that time. Up to his death, he never experienced any major health abnormalities I could associate with cancer signs. Malaria, headache, toothache, backache maybe as a result of too much bending during farming and eye problems were the constant health issues he regularly suffered from.

My mother, a wonderful woman, was always in very good mood. She was talkative to us as well as to other people in the various neighborhoods we stayed. She never worked but was a house wife taking care of the family. In the village, I recall seeing her waking up so early each morning to travel a long distance to the farm and return very late during hours of evenings often with a heavy load of harvest and firewood on her head. Just after reaching our hut, she always took a large container to go fetching water for drinking and to make a meal for us. After the meal, we always said and I remember this very well "Thank you mother." But, we realized that she was not happy because food in our plates was often completely finished; hence her worry that we were not full. The only time she expressed happiness and could say "thank you for what?" were moments when there was a leftover to eat as breakfast the following morning. After

45

the faming activities, she regularly cut trees to make charcoal for sale to raise income for our household basic needs particularly her children's school fees and to purchase other items such salt, oil and others for cooking. The daily pressure of the load she always carried on her head finally wiped out most of her hair making her a bold just as men. But, she always endured this to ensure we had food and went to school. As a result of this, her health rapidly deteriorated leading to her passing the other side at a very old age two years of her husband's death. Mother, I have tears in eyes and constantly dropping to the earth you tilled to provide food for us. I say many thanks to you. Similar health issues than those experienced by my father were also common for my mother during her lifetime. I never saw anything suspicious of signs which would have prompted me to conclude that she might have suffered from cancer at any time.

The first child in our family, a girl, became always sick after she was married and more so, after her first pregnancy. Unfortunately, she lost almost all her blood from hemorrhagic during the delivery but she survived. When she was discharged, she continued to be very sick and due to lack of resources in the family and proper health services in the village, she never received good health care. She passed away few days after leaving behind a girl baby child less than 1 month old. It was not a cancer. In the late hours of the evening the day she was buried—when we had just wished good night each other and lied on our sleeping place before even closing eyes—all of us clearly heard her voice requesting that we should bring the bible she has forgotten in the hut to her new place pointing out where the bible was and pleading that this needed to be placed on top of her new place. It was then that my mother arose and asked if we have heard that. Surprisingly, everyone said yes almost at the same time. Everyone had clearly heard my sister's voice. The mother went on crying again and again the whole night. In the morning, the father located the bible in her bag and we all went to her grave where the bible was deposited. We all left the place crying. My mother kept and continued providing maternal milk for the baby up to sometime she could feed on solid food. Since then up to her adulthood she remained in our household. Since I was so close to my sister, I made a vow to give her name to my first child regardless of the sex and to take care of her child when I complete my education. Fortunately after our wedding, we were blessed to have a girl as our first born. We named her after my sister's name and I took with me the child she left. However, she later returned to my parents' household when I travelled to US for graduate studies. At moment, she has her own two children and she is doing well in the village.

The third born child just after me, also a girl, died during her sixth year of life. Her death was caused by a severe infection following a traditional excision in the village of hernia using unsterilized razorblades. Beside intestine infection, she had also lost a considerable amount of blood during the procedure leading to a persistent anemia and development of malnutrition symptoms. As my parents were unable to afford suitable health services for her and supply in good time sustained nutritious foods to compensate for the lost blood and essential elements for body building, she became very ill. Her sickness—which lasted more than six months—was characterized by a considerable weight loss, loss of appetite, abdominal enlargement, hair shading and feet swelling. She passed away very young and for reasons she did not know but not from cancer. The remaining seven children – five gentlemen and two ladies – are alive and in good health. Among them, I am the only one who has suffered from cancer for the first time.

During my life up to the time I became devastated and weak due to the current illness, I have been actively engaged in a broader range of sporting activities all-over to enhance my functional capacity particularly during my university education period. I had mostly participated in playing football also called soccer by others even up to national and university competitions.

In every team I performed, I have been an outstanding middle field player always carrying the No. 6 jersey. I also played volleyball, went swimming when opportunities arose, and jogging and walking almost every day. By the way, in Africa where I come from, walking long distance every day is a common practice because of lack of own vehicle or scarcity of public transport. All these activities were much helpful in widening my personal friendships and strengthening my social interaction with other peers.

The foodstuffs I always ate are those which are commonly consumed by everyone in my tribe, clan, and family and others where I had been living throughout the country and abroad. The food habit I had inherited has been passed on from one generation to another and so, it has fully sustained my clan's continuity. My main staple is comprised of maize and cassava, which are processed into floor to make a consistent pasty porridge called "nshima or bidia" in my mother language—Luba—or also commonly known as "fufu" throughout the DR Congo. "Nshima" is popularly served with a wide range of relish including several indigenous vegetables (cassava, beans, pumpkins and sweetpotato leaves; mushrooms; okra; rape; cabbage; egg plants, amaranth; hibiscus, spinach and other several types of wild vegetables) and either meats (beef; pork; chicken; duck; rabbit, goat; and wild meats from rodents; antelopes; wild pigs; elephants; birds; monkeys; big reptiles etc.) or different types of fish (fresh, salted or smoked), and insects such as caterpillars, flying termites and grasshoppers. Many households in Africa consider forest and uncultivated savannah areas as locations where various animals can be traditionally hunted to derive numerous wildlife products such as bush meat that is an important source of protein. Hunters are mostly men who hunt for both subsistence and cash needs. Rice and plantains are also served to eat with the above relish. Other foods I have been consuming could also include sweetpotato, yams, cocoyams, groundnuts and beans to name but a few. The relish is mostly prepared using palm oil, which is rich in vitamin A, with condiments including tomato, onions and pepper. It is only occasionally when financial opportunities permit that some kinds of foods considered luxurious such as eggs, processed cereals, cheeses and salads are taken. The main meals have often been served once a day in the evening during the time I was in my young age in the village for my parents always left home in the early hours of morning going to the farm—the only source of our household's livelihood—and returned very late in the evening. Then, the mother had to rush to the spring located in the nearby gallery forest, about 1 km of distance, to fetch water to use for drinking and cooking. It is after that she could start making our meals. Often, the breakfast was the leftover from yesterday meals if this was available and western snacks, as we know them now a day, were nonexistent in between meals except on occasions when grilled or boiled cassava and sweetpotato tubers were eaten with groundnuts. However, at my adult age and now living in urban cities, I could afford three meals a day namely the breakfast, lunch and dinner, and in between snacks. These foods have been always also supplemented with the consumption of diverse fruits such as banana, papaya, avocado, oranges, mandarins, lemons, pineapple, sugarcane, mangustants, mango, guava, and several other types including numerous wild fruits. Certainly, I believe the nutritional compositions of our indigenous foods as well as the meals available in various towns have been adequate to provide for a substantive substrate that would sustain effectively one's living healthy physiological functions—growth, reproduction and productivity. In fact, I have rarely experienced illness for a very long past period until recently when my health began to deteriorate. I have always been in good health; thanks for the Lord's grace.

Though I have never tried it, men are known in my tribe as dogs' eaters. When a dog is identified as a pet, it is locally called "mbua." In this case, the dog is considered among the members of the household assisting for protection as well as for other numerous duties. However, it always happens that the owner and friends conspire to use it for food often by the end of year. Then, it changes to name to be called "chibelabela." They will go after it. They will catch, tight all the legs and slaughter it sometimes by pounding to death with sticks. "Chibelabela" is put into pieces of meat and cooked only by male normally once a year. Women are not allowed to approach the site of cooking for reasons I do not personally know. This is the current practice which is based on traditional beliefs. The cooking of dog meat is made using firewood and a pot which will usually be disposed of after it is served as dish. The meat is constantly stirred while boiling using sticks. Palm oil, salt, tomatoes, onion and a certain type of a wild vegetable called "chikota" are added to taste. Apparently, it is believed that eating the dog dish often brings strength.

As indicated early, many people in Africa—young, adults and seniors—die from various sicknesses some of which are of unknown diagnostic cause. It may be that cancer is part of the causes of so many human diseases in Africa. Parkin *et al.* (2003) reported that in Africa cancer cases can only be known when they come into contact with health services—hospitals, health centres, clinics and laboratories. In instances where households' income is constrained, access to health facilities by inhabitants became limited, so many of diseased people remain homes without health care. In such situation, they rely on numerous kinds of wild plants from forests including epiphytes, herbs, lianas and trees, and different parts of plants such as roots, barks, leaves, flowers and fruits for medicinal formulas often prescribed by traditional healers as traditional medicines to cure the diseases.

Moreover, I have passed a large part of my life in the coppebelt mining areas both in southern DR Congo and north-western Zambia. In these locations, effluents from mineral extractions by mining companies found deliberately their way in rivers contaminating agricultural lands, food crops and products, rivers and water tables with heavy metals such as manganese (Mn), nickel (Ni), lead (Pb), zinc (Zn), cobalt (Co), arsenic (As), uranium (U), cadmium (Cd) and copper (Cu) etc. The presence of these metals in food or water to drink is hazardous to human health and may result in several diseases including cancer. WHO (2007) recognized arsenic as one of the few carcinogenic chemicals that contaminate drinking water around the world and provided recommendations with clear guidelines for provision of a good quality drinking water for the population (www.who.int/water sanitation health/dwq/arsenic). Several other safety standards for toxic chemicals in food, including carcinogenic contaminants such as heavy metals and mycotoxins have also been provided by FAO and WHO (FAO/WHO, 1993; 2001 and WHO, 2009).

Personally, I love eating mushrooms mainly because of their appealing taste. Mushrooms growing in these polluted ecological zones of copperbelt, where the land is continuously contaminated by a wide variety of pollutants from mining waste, are known to rapidly absorb heavy metals into their tissues and by doing so, they clean the environment or can be used to reclaim degraded lands (Bressa et al., 1988; Stijve and Roschnik, 1974; Stijve, 1992; Overstorey, 2004). The most amazing dietetic value of edible mushrooms is that they are very rich in protein and are an excellent source of fibre, vitamins, and several other minerals. Their high protein content makes them an ideal food because they contain all the amino acids essential to human nutrition. Mushrooms are also a cholesterol-free food. They can prevent atherosclerosis due to their high fibre content (Ingram, 2002) as well as cure heart diseases (Sikombwa and Piearce, 1985). Similarly, there have been various claims about the immune-modulatory effects of mushroom lentinan compound in human (Dawn Soo, 2002), although these have not yet shown any significance in a therapeutic context per se. Suggestions that these effects could account for the demonstrated anti-bacterial and anti-viral action have considerably risen, and constitute currently an exciting prospect, especially in the face of a post-antibiotic era and the wake of an increasing incidence of HIV/AIDS in the world.

As a Plant Pathologist, I often also handle different types of plant- and food- contaminating microorganisms for my field and laboratory work without appropriate protection measures like gloves and mouth masks. Some of these germs, particularly species of moldy fungi commonly found in food commodities during drying and in storage, can produce mycotoxins including aflatoxin, fumonisin, ochratoxin and many others (Marasas *et al.*, 1977; Williams *et al.*, 1994; Leslie, 2005) that are known to cause a number of human diseases including cancer (Williams *et al.*, 1994; Miller and Marasas, 2002). Were all these the possible causes that led to the development of this colorectal cancer into my body? When exactly the illness was initiated within my colon? These are just some of the few questions I asked myself but without any clear answer in mind.

Sharing diagnostic results with friends

To discharge myself from the stress and continuous emotion following the illness diagnosis, I discussed with my spouse if I could reach out and share the outcome of the diagnostic with other friends. I considered it unhealthy living with the burden of emotions in isolation, hence wanted them to be more close to me in this harsh time I was going through the agony of my life. Indeed, I felt so relieved when I had communicated about it to friends. I wrote an electronic mail which I copied to many of them to let them know my health situation and why I was in Canada. My letter read:

Dear friends,

Greetings from Canada. I felt I should inform you that I left suddenly Zambia last April 2011 very sick. I could not eat, do toilet, walk, speak and open my eyes. All the way I was assisted by immigration officers and flight attendants and everyone wondered how they allowed me enter the plane to Canada. Upon arrival at Ottawa airport, was taken out on wheelchair and my spouse took me straight to the hospital. After a lot of examinations and tests, I was diagnosed with the colon-rectal cancer at stage 3 towards 4. At this stage often the patient is sent back home to die but luckily enough one of the Medical Doctor came to see me late in the night and consented to take me for various treatments. I was admitted and went in for the first surgery to redirect the colon into an artificial push, anus as colostomy through the belly to allow me evacuate my bowl. Then I undergone radiation combined with the chemotherapy treatment for about 4 weeks to reduce the tumor size. Later I went in again for the major surgery that took 9 hours to remove it as it had already spread to other organs. The colostomy was changed to ileostomy to allow the reversal at a later stage. Now I am again following a high dose of chemotherapy which will go up to June-July after which another operation will be made to reverse the stoma. It has been very difficult considering the various side effects of the treatments but, I have to endure them because I came to receive treatments to save my life. The support of my family and other friends has been considerable especially the fatigue and emotion we are going through as well as the cost for medical interventions (Doctors' consultations, different tests such as MRI, CT scan, X-ray and ultra-sound ect.). Luckily, the government of Canada, through its Ministry of Health, is taking care of most of my expenditure. Please inform other members of our group and colleagues so that everyone could pray for my recovery. Muimba-Kankolongo

Surprisingly, the responses I got back were amazing. Fewer of the encouraging feedback messages I received included the following.

They wrote:
Thursday, August 4, 2011
Dear Dr Kankolongo

It has been a while since you left Kitwe to Canada for treatment. I hope that all is well with regards the procedures, you have to go through, as briefed by Dr Mwitwa. I just want to tell you that you are in my prayers for a speedy recovery. I miss you so much and looking forward to your coming back. Greetings to the family. Phil. Ng'andwe.

Monday, March 19, 2012
Dear Muimba,

Your message arrives as quite a shock. I cannot imagine what you and your family have endured for more than the past year and continuing. Your message is also one of hope. That the therapy is doing its healing work and the prospect that the doctors may be able to reverse the stoma is our strong hope. For starters, Fran and I will pray for your steady and complete recovery and the wellbeing of your family. I will share your message with as many of your Cornell colleagues as I have contact info for. You have many friends. I expect some of your friends will ask how they can help in addition to prayer. Is there a medical fund set up to receive donations to help with your expenses? Any instructions of where to send donations and how checks should be made out? What is your apartment address and phone number in Canada? Thank you so much for writing to me. I admire you very much. Keep fighting to regain your health. Please say hi your family and stay in touch. You are in our thoughts, Gary and Fran

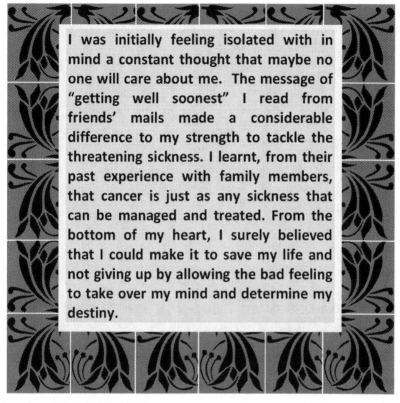

I was initially feeling isolated with in mind a constant thought that maybe no one will care about me. The message of "getting well soonest" I read from friends' mails made a considerable difference to my strength to tackle the threatening sickness. I learnt, from their past experience with family members, that cancer is just as any sickness that can be managed and treated. From the bottom of my heart, I surely believed that I could make it to save my life and not giving up by allowing the bad feeling to take over my mind and determine my destiny.

Monday, March 19, 2012
Dear Muimba,

Gary told me about your challenging fight with cancer. I am so sorry to hear this. I am very familiar with colon-rectal cancer as my father got this disease (it was found early with my dad and he is still healthy at age 89) as well as a close friend of mine here in Madison (who is not doing well). I know this is an incredible drain on your energy and finances as well as the impact on your family. I will pray for you and your family. Let me know if there is any way I can help you, Sincerely,

Nancy Keller, Professor

Saturday, March 31, 2012
Hello Muimba,

Gary informed us of all the pain you have endured over the past year with cancer. I cannot imagine how difficult it has been. But you are strong, and we are all praying for you. I have sent you a letter, it should be there in two weeks I hope. I would like to come visit you if it's okay and you are able to have visitors. Let me know if and when this will be okay. Best, Denis A. Shah, Ph.D.

Tuesday, May 8, 2012
Dear Muimba,

I received a call from Gary Bergstrom which brought me both the good news that you are in Canada and the not good news that you have been extremely ill. I hope that you are definitely on the improvement and that you will turn the corner on battling the cancer. It is fortunate that you have survived to this point---you are clearly both very tough and determined. And your family is clearly trying to do its part. Please know that you are in our family's best wishes and prayers. Please do stay in contact with us. I have passed the news on to my daughters and perhaps you will hear from Martha and Jesse at some point. When I return to Oregon (I am working in Virginia for two weeks while Miriam took her 2nd year of law finals; it helps to have help with the children during that time), I will send on our annual greeting to you which will bring you up to date on our family activities. All are well although my own sister had surgery for two different cancers last year (colon and breast) so I am now being even more vigilant about my own health. Please take care. Our love to you and your family, Stella Melugin Coakley

My reply to all those who wrote for their encouraging and comforting words was as follow:

Dear friends,

Thank you so very much for your prompt response and I also receive a message from Nancy. It took so long to write to friends like you thinking this message will very much disturb their morale but am happy you received it well with a great enthusiasm. I will continue updating you on the progress of my health. There is no anything like a medical fund we have set rather than asking friends to put me and the family in prayer during this hard time. It is very hard but we have faith in the Lord that it will come to pass. One of the Doctors told me during a visit that I will have to take each day as a day, which I do. In case colleagues want to assist, I will be willing to provide them with my account No. Our home address is 1070 Candlewood street, Orleans, On K4A 5E9 and our home telephone No. is (613)-837-3504. Once again,

thank you very much. Muimba-Kankolongo

CHAPTER V

A BYPASSING COLOSTOMY

> *The cancerous tumor—already in stage 3 to 4—caused total obstruction of the rectal channel making me unable to pass the stool through the anus and had invaded several organs including possibly the seminal vesicles.*

owards the end of May 2011, the admission department from the Civic Hospital, which is also part of the Ottawa General Hospital, called that a surgery is now planned to open up the obstructed anal channel with a defunctionalized colostomy. This will allow for a free bowel movement through the artificial opening and reduce the abdomen swelling, pain and discomfort. I was briefed about all necessary pre- and post-surgery procedures to prepare well for the surgery. The information included what to do during the evening before the day of the surgery and the morning of the surgery before going to the hospital as well as at the surgical day care unit, in the operating room and after surgery in the post-anesthetic care unit. Similarly, I was provided with details dealing with various visits by medical doctors, care I will receive in the hospital inpatient room and at home after I am discharged from the hospital. Prior to the surgery, some tests were conducted to determine again characteristics and the exact stage of the tumor.

Endoscopy

About two days before the procedure, I signed the consent document for the procedure after related risks and benefits were explained. I was also prescribed some laxatives to take and requested to eat a minimal food and drink lots of water to clear the bowel so that a clear view of the colon and rectum linings could be seen throughout the surgery. Specifically, the preparation for the test consisted of halting any medications such as aspiring and for blood thinning a week before the procedure; and taking the bowel preparing medications—two packets of Pico Salax or Colyte and 4 Dulcolax tablets—as prescribed. A slight meal could be taken in the morning of the procedure day and then remain on clear fluids or some few sips of water up to 3 hours before the operation. In the endoscopy suite, I was anesthetized before the colonoscope was introduced through the anus all the way to the hepatic flexure.

Magnetic Resonance Imaging (MRI)

The test uses a magnetic field through a scanner that sends out radio waves to the body which are reflected back to produce 3-dimensional pictures which are processed using a computer system (National Cancer Institute, 2013). Before the procedure, a gadolinium substance that collects around the cancerous cells was intravenously injected into my body to allow for brighter and clear images during observation. The tumor (Figs. 8&9) is mid-rectum circumferential about 8.5 cm from the anal verge and extending for approximately 9.8 cm with possible bilaterally infiltration of the seminal vesicles and the right pelvic sidewall. It was causing large bowel obstruction with a very significant proximal fecal loading. More than five lymph nodes—receptors of some drainage from intestinal tracts and out of abdominal organs—were observed in the rectosigmoid mesentery (region of the descending colon) and behind the abdominal cavity in the retroperitoneum or upper side of the rectum as well as in the lower left external inguinal region (iliac region) with the largest nodea being 18 mm.

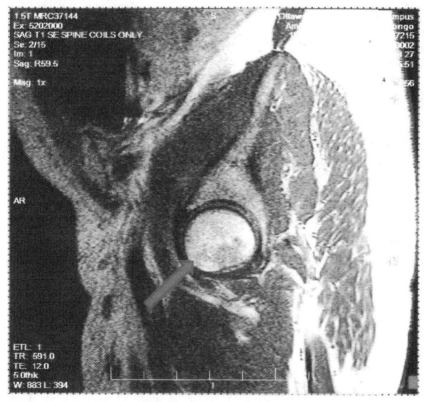

Figure 8. Left side MRI image of the cancerous tumor extending from the anal verge to infiltration of seminal vesicles

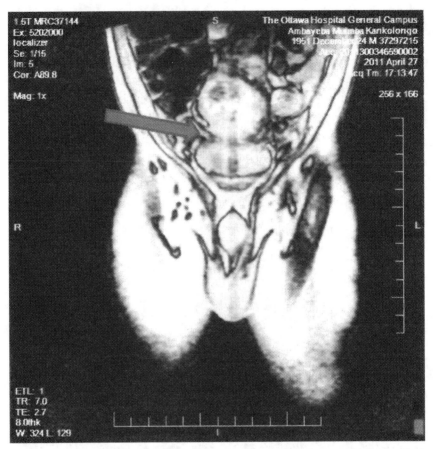

Figure 9. MRI image in sapine position of the tumor in my pelvis causing considerable bowel obstruction

Physical examinations

From the examination by both the chemotherapy and radiation oncologists, it was clear that I was looking slightly well although the continuous suffering of constipation with only a liquefied stool coming out. Results of my blood analysis revealed that I was also iron deficient. However, the acute pain I was initially feeling was now controlled with the hydromorphone drug but there was still intermittent pain coming from the right inguinal area. The chest was clear, the heart sound normal and the abdomen soft and nontender. The rectal examination showed an empty rectum. However, because of signs of imminent obstruction of the colon from the developing tumor, it was recommended that I should have a diverting colostomy and be urgently referred to the surgeon for the operation. During subsequent visits and discussions with the radiation and chemotherapy Oncologists in the surgical inpatient service following other symptoms of overflow diarrhea from a partial bowel obstruction I presented, it was finally decided that adjuvant chemotherapy and radiation and surgery to remove the rectal tumor and enlarged lymph nodes were suggested as the only potentially aggressive and curative treatments for my sickness. They proposed that I should be administered intravenously an additional chemotherapy medication consisting of an infusional 5-fluorouracil (5-FU) post-surgery of tumor removal. During the meeting, various side effects of chemotherapy regiment concomitantly administered with radiation treatment were also clearly stated. They included effects like nausea, loss of appetite, body itching, hair shading and most importantly the possibility of affecting the nerve systems around the pelvis and in legs. Complications that might ensue from the surgery as well as more usual things such as dehydration, general body fatigue, skin changes and other malaise were also discussed. But, they indicated that all the specific surgery details will be given to me by the surgeon who will perform the operation in due time.

Surgery

I signed the informed consent form for the surgery at the Civic Hospital and discussed further risks and benefits of the intervention with the surgeon. Two weeks before the surgery, my blood was collected for laboratory analysis to establish the haemoglobin level. In addition, the surgery protocol was followed on that day. In the evening and morning before the exact date, I was instructed to take bath using a regular soap and also to wash my hair, always avoiding scented products. I had to stop eating solid food at least the night before the surgery, but I could drink at least two cups of colorless drinks such as water, apple juice, sprite, ginger ale, 7-Up etc. Before going to the hospital for the operation, I could take my usual blood pressure and other vitamin medications, and do all necessary toiletings but avoiding perfume, scented lotions, aftershave, and hair products and wear loose and comfortable clothes.

I reported to the Surgical Day Care Unit of the hospital at 8h00 am. After the secretary checked my identification from the computer, I was told to remove all my cloth and wear a gown and to wait for the nurse in a room. About 30 minutes later, I was called and taken to one of the operating rooms in a stretcher. When we arrived by the door of the room but still in the hall, I asked the nurse to give me the urinal as I sensed like passing the urine before going in. She presented me with one and left to hand in my file to other nurses already inside. I tried to urinate but could not. When she returned, she pointed out that there was nothing in the container. I knew, she said, it was a normal fearful reaction for all patients before the surgery. Then she gave me a plastic hat to cover the head, wished me good luck for the surgery and left. Another nurse from the room joined me outside to record my health history particularly if I had in the past experienced heart attack or stroke and collect additional information including whether I am allergic to any medications and if I smoke or take alcohol. Finally, she asked if I understood the procedure they were about to perform.

Thereafter, I was taken inside and this was my first time to enter a surgical room. Generally, it is very clean room, well maintained in sterile conditions, and brightly lit and maintained in cooler environmental conditions. There were two nurses taking the inventory of tools in one corner while the other two to the next corner were connecting various machines including monitors of the vital signs. The anesthesiologist and one nurse were standing by the stretcher. All were wearing sterile protecting gowns and gloves as well as shoe covers, masks, caps, eye shields, and other coverings to prevent the spreading of germs particularly when talking. They helped me move from the stretcher to a narrow operating room table which has safety straps to keep the patient in a good position and covered me with a warm blanket to keep my body warm and comfortable before the surgery. The anesthesiologist explained that he will carry out an intravenous infusion of the sedation anesthesia to put me to sleep during the operation. Up to this time I was very much awake and I have not seen the surgeon.

Electrical cables connected to the monitoring equipment were applied onto my thoracic area for the assessment of my vital signs whereas a blood pressure cuff was put on one of my arms to follow it during the operation. Similarly, electrodes were placed on my chest to monitor my heart beat, and the oxygen mask placed over my mouth and nose and a probe on one of the fingers to measure the blood oxygen level. There were also huge circular sets of bright lamps in the ceiling. Finally, I was told that the anesthetic infusion was now going to be given. I still never saw the surgeon up to this time. Before I was put to sleep, I said rapidly and quietly my prayer to The LORD telling Him that;

> "He is the Healer and the Provider of intelligence to anyone including physicians and nurses in the room." I closed eyes lost in confession pleading to The Almighty for his Hands. Dear LORD, I said, I pray for your hand and grace during this surgery. In the holy name of Your Son Jesus Christ I pray that the surgery goes on well and for your guidance to the surgeon during the intervention."

After I said Amen! I did not know what followed next as I was as deep asleep. It is until I was awakened in the post-anesthetic care unit (PACU) that another nurse said to me the surgery is now over and that I have a colostomy in place in the abdominal area (Fig. 10). By then, the surgeon had already informed my spouse in the waiting area about the completion of the surgery and my returning to the recovery room in good conditions without any complications related to the surgery.

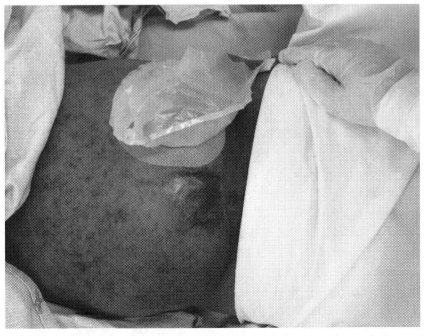

Figure 10. A colostomy bag inserted on the left side of my abdomen to allow diverting the stool from the anus.

The surgeon described that beside the general anesthesia, I also received antibiotics prior to the surgery after I was sterilely prepared, draped in the usual sterile fashion and kept lying on the back also known as dorsal or supine position for the surgery. The team made first a short incision inside the umbilicus, opened the fascia under direct vision and inserted a 12 mm trocar—to allow for subsequent placement of other instruments such as graspers, scissors, staplers, etc. and a 10 mm scope inside the abdomen creating the presence of air or gas in the abdominal (peritoneal) cavity (a pneumoperitoneum) of about 15 mm Hg. It is then that they could have a good observation of the inside of the abdomen. They did not notice any further invasion of the cancer to other organs, but rather the mass was in the pelvic area. In addition, there was no lesion on the liver although they noticed some enlargement of the small and large bowels. They inserted other 5 mm trocars in the left lower quadrant and found the sigmoid colon that they easily butted on the skin where there was the stoma mark that was initially done by the nurse. A circular incision of the skin was made down to the fascia which was opened in a cross form using the heating of tissues with electricity or electrocautery. They then opened the muscle and the longitudinal plane parallel to the rectus muscle to enter the abdomen. At this point, they easily grasped and pulled the bowel through the incision and finally closed the umbilical incision and the 5 mm port incision making sure there was no twist in the mesentery of the bowel.

A red latex tube was placed under the stoma before opening it and then fixed it to the abdominal wall using interrupted stitches of Maxon No. 2-0. This was then fixed to the skin also using interrupted stitches of Maxon in the total plane in the bowel and on the dermis. The colostomy appliance was put on and the stoma was warmed and well tolerated at the end of the procedure. During the procedure, I lost approximately 50 mL of blood. Generally, a stoma is created by bringing a portion of the inner layer of the small or large bowel out through a surgical-created opening in the abdomen (Convatec, 2009). The surgeon released me from the operating room to the recovery room in good condition without complications.

When I woke up and fully recovered my conscience, I realized I was no longer in the surgery room rather in an open area with several other patients in other beds. I was still connected to an oxygen supply line and a nurse, wearing normal nursing clothes, was by my bed side recording my vital signs (blood pressure, temperature from the ear, and heart bits and sounds). She said the procedure, which went well, finished few minutes ago. Then she asked if I was feeling some pain and where on the body I was in pain. She also requested that I open my mouth, cough at least twice or three times and respire deeply in and out. At that time I could feel some intermittent pain around the surgery wound but not as acute as what I was experiencing prior to the operation. She gave me some pain killer tablets to prevent and manage it, and continued monitoring my vital signs and recording my temperature until a room was identified and made ready for me in the inpatient ward upstairs. In addition, she monitored the flow of liquid-like stools in the colostomy pouch and cleaned it. Shortly after, I was transferred to my room in the inpatient ward.

Colostomy

Though the surgery relieved me from the acute abdominal pain I was previously experiencing, I was however sad due to the presence of a permanent colostomy that I will have to bear the rest of my life. Stool and gas will no longer be eliminated through the anus rather will now pass through the stoma to the pouch which is attached on my abdomen. Because it does not have a sphincter muscle like in our body, I will also lack a voluntary control over bowel movements. In the ward, nurses trained me how to manage the colostomy; that is when it should be clear mainly when it is one third to about one half full, how to clean it, when a new one should be replaced after rinsing the skin around with water and drying it before a new one is applied, and how to activate the adhesive by holding it against the body for few seconds. When it is time to change shifts, the next nurse always introduced herself or himself to me.

"Hi or Hello!"
H/she often said....
"My name is ....,"
"I will be your nurse and will take care of you for the following hours."
"How are you feeling today?"
"Any pain?"

When he or she says so, they really mean it. They regularly checked on me and often made sure I was comfortably well without any signs of pain. They also checked on the bowel movement and the breathing sound. Initially, they assisted to my move to get out of the bed to reach the bathroom or use the bedpan or urinal when necessary, and access the bedside table where they put food and drink (fresh water or juice), the bell to use any time I need assistance and the light switch. They also assisted on the move on the bed like sitting at the side, performing exercise of the ankles and leg pumping, deep breathing and coughing, and sitting in the chair to walking in the halls. Before bed time, they always inject the patient with anticoagulant drug either on the abdomen or limb. Thereafter, they gradually let me do everything alone as the recovery from the surgery advances. Finally, they also provided on time the medications as prescribed by physicians. More importantly, they ensured hands were always clean before doing anything on the patient and thereafter when they are through.

From a liquid diet following the surgery (Fig. 11) to allow the digestive system adjust to the new artificial system; I slowly resumed eating the normal solid food as I recovered from the operation and my system readjusts to this type of foods. The foods taken in the hospital were carefully selected to avoid, at least during the first days to about six to eight weeks following the surgery, those with high fiber and residue content first to see how well the system could tolerate them and also to avoid such problems as cramping, diarrhea, nausea and vomiting. These had to be eaten slowly taking small bites at times and chewing them completely before swallowing to decrease fecal output, reduce irritation in the stomach and avoid unexpected potential obstruction. For fruits, I had to remove the skin, seeds and the membranes. Booklets on nutritional guidelines outlining what to eat and what to avoid were provided with the view to help control or prevent obstructions, and control the frequency of bowel movements. As supplement, intake of Ensure Plus calories and Boost drinks were highly recommended because of their complete and well balanced nutrition content. These are good source of protein; vitamins and numerous minerals that could help with the body building and maintaining of a healthy weight rapidly.

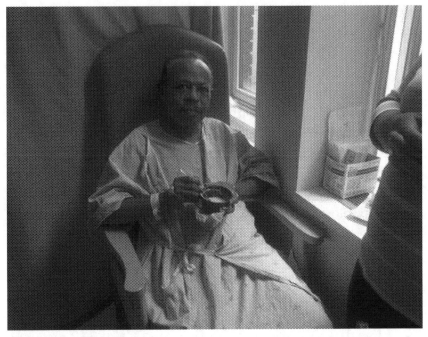

Figure 11. At the Riverside Hospital on a liquid diet after surgery for the bypassing colostomy

Follow up post-colostomy surgery tests

Various tests were again performed following the surgery when I developed high fever. It was found that I had considerable increase in white blood cell count and suspicion was of possibly pneumonia infection. However, they found that my lungs were clear, the lining of the heart sac or the cardiomediastinal silhouete was within normal limits and that there was no evidence of pneumonia. A CT scan of the abdomen and pelvis with intravenous contrast was again performed and revealed that my liver was within the normal size with a normal contour and homogenous structure. On the biliary tree—the path by which bile is secreted by the liver then transported to the first part of the small intestine and the gallbladder which is small organ where bile is stored before it is released into the small intestine—was partially distented with no evidence, however, of any foreign bodies like intraluminal radiodense calculi. The bile ducts were not dilated. The pancreas was in normal shape and there were no intrapancreatic duct dilatation or peripancreatic fluid. The stomach was partially distended with some material, likely ingested food, within the left portion of the stomach's body or stomach fundus that allows for an accumulation of gases produced by chemical digestion. Small bowel loops were nondistended and there was no evidence of fat stranding to suggest any inflammation. On the pelvis, in the rectosigmoid area, there was still that large enhancing mass measuring about 11.0 x 7.0 cm (longitudinal x transverse dimensions), an increase from the previously observed size of 9.3 x 3.0 cm. But unfortunately, there was a clear evidence of further spread of the mass with regional stranding surrounding mesenteric fat—visceral fat in the close proximity to the portal circulation, affecting directly the liver, which is the main regulator of body metabolic homeostasis—and no evidence of infected fluid collection that would suspect the presence of an abscess.

Furthermore, there was no evidence of colonic obstruction although the colon was severely loaded with fecal material. There were also multiple enlarged lymph nodes in front of the lumbar bodies near the aorta or the para-aortic and aortocaval regions and in the common iliac area but bilaterally. The adrenal glands were normal and there was a moderate right-sided distention of both the ureter and the renal pelvis and calices or hydoureteronephrosis on the kidneys with the ureter being distended up to level of the rectosigmoid mass. The right side kidney appeared to be in external compression from the large pelvic mass, which could not exclude completely the involvement by the tumor in the urinary tract. The urinary bladder was minimally distended and the prostate was within its normal size. After reviewing the scan, the oncologist felt it was comfortable to treat me for the tumor and the lymph nodes using first the radiation therapy. All team members of physicians agreed that the radiation treatment be given to me as planned. Unfortunately while I was still admitted in the hospital after the colostomy operation, I was found to be infected with some bacteria which have translocated throughout a large portion of the abdominal system. As a curative measure, I was injected with the antibiotic ceftriaxone/flagyl and given another one, clavulin, on the discharge day to be orally taken at home.

Physical examinations of the abdomen and colostomy on the day to leave the hospital showed that I was doing well and the stoma was pink, healthy and working well. The colostomy was high enough out of the field where the radiation treatment would not reach. Both the radiation and chemotherapy oncologists were then ready for the administration of a curative therapy with neoadjuvant chemoradiation treatment, using a continuous infusion of 5-FU as initially suggested, whereby the lymph nodes will be included at the L4 level in the large field. I did not have any fever and my abdomen was soft and nontender.

Discharge and setback

Every morning while in the hospital, resident doctors visited to check on patients. When they enter the room, always in company of medical students and/or visiting doctors, they greeted you and asked some questions particularly to know as how the patient was doing, how he slept, and if he or she had some pain and where on the body it was paining. At times, they performed physical examinations and requested if there was something of concern they should know. If necessary, they also prescribed appropriate medications to manage your concern. Seven days later after hospitalization, I was discharged after a complete assessment by the physiotherapist. The nurse provides assessment in regards to pain management, increase movement and mobility, restoration of function and on the education. Specifically, she wanted to ensure I was able to walk and climb stairs by myself and without difficulty; correctly pronounce some specific words, answer correctly to some questions like dates and times of the year, and where the patient was before being released from the hospital. Before leaving the hospital, necessary arrangements were made for follow ups with home care nurses through the Community

Care Access Center (CCAC). A one day's notice is given before the date of discharge so that you can be prepared and be ready to go back home. On the day of discharge and when it is after 10.00 am when waiting for transportation, I was moved out to the patient lounge to wait from there and allow nurses to prepare the room for other patients. My spouse drove me safely home without any major problem.

Three days following the discharge while at home, I noticed an abnormal swelling around the colostomy. I pulled out the pouch and realised the intestine was coming out as a result of colostomy prolapse. The suture ruptured making the intestine to be pushed out reaching about the knee level. I called and showed this to my spouse who quickly called the ambulance. Paramedics helped me to walk slowly to the ambulance where I was assisted to lie on my back on the bed. I was secured on it before being embarked in and rapidly drove to the Civic hospital emergency department. My third son was following the ambulance up to the hospital where we arrived within a few minutes. I was taken out and the stretcher was pushed in the corridor where I waited for about 15-25 minutes after which I was rushed to the operating room for a repair of the prolapsed loop colostomy.

Another surgeon with assistance from two other medical doctors led the operation. The general anesthesia and endotracheal intubation were carried out prior to their intervention. Then, the abdomen was well washed and sterilized before I was draped in the usual sterile fashion. They realised that the loop colostomy in the left lower quadrant was prolapsed and was like without any blood or ischemic looking. They managed to partially reduce its size while I was sleeping. The redundant bowel was cut back through an incision around the stoma and by separating the stoma at the site where my skin and the mucous membrane were merging or the mucocutaneous junction. The resection was about 10 cm of the sigmoid colon with sequential clamping, dividing and ligating the mesentery and then amputating the bowel with GIA-80 staplers. Upon examination of the remaining stoma, it was found that the two ends of the bowel that were bought out onto the surface of the abdomen or mucous fistula was intact with no evidence of prolapse in that area. As a result of this observation, they proceeded with the staple line amputation and the resewing of the end colostomy circumferentially to the skin edges using interrupted No. 3-0 Vicryl suture. A stoma appliance was then affixed at the end of the operation when they counted all sponges and instruments they used. After the operation, I was again transferred to the recovery room and then to my inpatient room where I stayed for seven additional days. As usual, the blood was regularly taken in the morning of each day for analysis. Unfortunately, the result of my blood analysis was still revealing bacterial infection. I was administered intravenously an antibiotic medication followed by an oral intake of another antibiotic for 10 days. By the discharge day, I was doing well.

While in the hospital and to avoid further suture rupture, nurses provided additional training about moving, positioning and getting out of bed as prescribed by the hospital (here reproduced with permission from the Department of Patient Advocacy; Ottawa Hospital, 2010). The emphasized was on always supporting the abdomen with either a pillow or any blanket during any movement on or from the bed such as bending knees and rolling from side to the back. Before leaving the bed, the nurse indicated to roll first on the side bringing knees up towards the abdomen. Then, placing upper hand on the bed below the elbow and raising the upper body off the bed by pushing down on the bed using the hand. After that, I had to swing my feet and legs over the bed's edge at the same time trying to bring the body to a sitting position. Once in this position, I should take a few seconds but also making sure I was in good balance before standing. At this point, I was requested to slowly slide my bottom to the edge of the bed and standing up with my back in a straight position. At the end of what I needed to accomplish when I left the bed, I had to reverse the process when I am ready to return into the bed.

CHAPTER VI
TUMOR SHRINKAGE

I was first administered an adjuvant radiation-chemotherapy regiment to shrink the tumor. During this period, I suffered from various side effects including nausea; some vomiting; a bit loss of appetite due to dry mouth and sore making food tasteless; partial hair loss; body itching mainly in the eyes which had become so dry; skin rash over my extremities, trunk and face; tingling of hand palms and feet soles; loss of sensation to touch particularly when it is cold; skin burn becoming darkish particularly on the face and the arm around where the treatment was infused; general fatigue and weakness; and numbness in feet, toes and fingers.

*A*s I indicated earlier, a chemo-radiation regiment followed by a surgery to remove the rectal tumor and enlarged lymph nodes and then a long cycle adjuvant chemotherapy were considered as potentially aggressive and curative treatments for my sickness. However, during appointments and discussions with various physicians including the oncologists I expressed my strong resolve for them to treat me aggressively to end the disease considering the severe pain and emotional death risk I was going through. Though they understood well my emotion and highly considered my feeling, they always tended to bring to the fore my awareness of the numerous risks that might ensue from an aggressive treatment such as this. On my side, I was mentally and physically well prepared to endure any treatment effects and surgical challenges.

Before treatments began, several meetings with doctors were scheduled for my health assessment. During each visit, I had to fill in and submit first to my patient designed nurse (PDN) a symptom assessment form. This was done using the computer evaluation program—Interactive Symptom Assessment And Collection (ISAAC) scale which provides for the overall review of cancer patients' feeling based on nine of the most common symptoms that they are experiencing. The scale for symptoms ranges from 0 = least to 10 = worse. It also assessed the level at which the patient's feeling has interfered with his or her normal daily activity. The activity includes such things like the general mood, walking capability, normal work (house, outside home) and relations with others, sleep and life enjoyment). The parameters assessed are level of pain, tiredness, shortness of breath, drowsiness, nausea, lack of appetite, depression, anxiety and overall wellbeing. Level of activity undertaking and their functions are also evaluated. The program is activated by swiping first the magnetic strip of one's health card on the indicated place in the computer and second by writing own password. Then, a computer screen prompts showing the 9 different potential symptoms for each of the health issue to be scored for. By keying in your assessment score on a specific circle, it changes the color indicating acceptance and that you should continue with the assessment of the following health issue and so on up to the end. At this point the program summarizes all the patient's scores for review after which you type the "Done touch" key to complete the assessment and print the form. After answering the nine requested questions, the final results are printed and these are submitted to the nurse. Using this chart, doctors will be updated with patient's feeling each time they meet them.

Oncologists recommended various tests to be performed prior to the treatments including examination of the chest, postoperative CT scan of the abdomen and pelvis with intravenous contrast and laboratory analysis of the colon specimen. It was found from these tests that lungs were normal and that there was neither any evidence of pneumonia nor other significant changes observed compared to findings from the previous chest examination. The chest showed clear lungs and the lining sac for the heart was within normal limits. The bones and soft tissues were also normal. The CT scan images showed that the liver had its normal size in contour with a homogenous structure. There was no suspicious solid nodule being identified. Moreover, bile ducts were not dilated and there was no other wall thickening although the gallbladder was partially distended. The pancreas was in normal shape and there was neither duct dilatation in the pancreas nor a collection of infected fluid around the pancreas. The stomach was partially distended while small bowel loops were nondistended with no evidence of fat stranding which could suggest any inflammatory changes. The interval diversion colostomy, which was lately performed on the left lower body quadrant, appeared to be within normal limits.

Although there was no any evidence of intra-abdominal abscess or perforation and any spread of the enlargement of lymphatic nodes or metastatic adenopathy on the pelvis around the rectosigmoid area, there was still that large enhancing mass of the tumor with approximately 11 x 7 cm (longitudinal x transverse dimensions), increasing from the prior size of 9.3 x 3 cm. While there was a clear evidence of its transoral spread with regional stranding around the mesenteric fat, no colonic obstruction was detected although there was a severely fecal loaded colon. Multiple enlarged lymph nodes were seen in the para-aortic and aortcaval regions which are in front of the lumbar vertebra to the lower border of the twelfth thoracic vertebra. Adrenal glands were all normal. At the right kidney, the ureter was distended up to the level of the tumor and this suggested that it might be in the external compression from the large pelvic mass and that the urinary tract involvement by the tumor could not be completely excluded. The bladder was minimally distended, but the prostate was in normal size. Based on these results, Oncologists agreed to start as soon as possible the radiation and chemotherapy treatments to shrink the tumor for the feasibility of the surgery to remove it.

Radiation

Before being subjected to the radiation, I went through a training program followed by an orientation of the various facilities and places where I will visit during its course. The training was centered on some topics that could help patients and their families understand the disease and how it can be treated, how the treatments work, their side effects and how these can be managed. Moreover, it is planned for patients to know diverse emotional and social challenges they might encounter and to prepare them for a good recovery. Surprisingly for me, I realized that the disease was just as any other disease that affects human being only until we went, my spouse and I, for the first visit through the various facilities of the regional cancer center at the Ottawa General Hospital. We came across many people of different sexes, ages, ethnic and cultural backgrounds, and education in the lounges waiting for either consultation with physicians or for treatment of the cancer disease. Instantly, the overwhelming distress I had and the sadness which had surrounded me for several months disappeared. I felt strength to carry on after realizing I was not alone but several other people had a similar disease and were going through identical pains and emotions as I was. After the training, I was comfortably well prepared and strong enough to go through with the treatments because I was aware of what to expect at this time.

The radiation treatment was scheduled to commence at the beginning of July 2011 and be administered daily for 4 and half weeks. Prior to the treatment, the blood test needed to be done to check on the counts of both white cells and haemoglobin. Generally, if these are low the treatment may be delayed because of considerable weakness, tiredness, dizziness and sometimes headache and shortness of breath the treatment can cause. Since the results of my blood work were good, the examination of the abdomen and colostomy perfect and the review of the CT scan images adequate, the Oncologists were now comfortable that I start the treatment. I was required to report for it to the radiation wing.

Radiation therapy also known as local therapy due to its targeting of only a specific part of the body usually the pelvic area, uses X-rays to kill the tumor or, if given over several weeks in small doses, it results in a decline of the affected cells. In the radiation room, I met two technicians who assisted in my lying down on my back on the table directly under the radiation machine. They covered any unwanted body areas with bed sheets to protect them from irradiation. Then, one marked first places where the rays will be directed and both of them adjusted the radiation beam of the X-ray machine to direct the rays to the area of interest on my body. Thereafter, they went out to another room to start the machine and monitor the rays delivery through a computer, which took only a few minutes as the machine moved around my body.

My Oncologist, a radiation specialist, made a clearly thought plan that I first go through some treatments including the radiation and chemotherapy to reduce the tumor size before any attempt to remove it. This was the best approach in tackling my sickness.

Chemotherapy

Concomitant with the radiation, I was also administered a chemotherapy treatment as per recommendations of my Oncologist. I was informed that the chemotherapy drugs will slow or stop cancerous cells from growing, multiplying or spreading to other parts of the body and can also shrink tumors. Its only problem is that it affects the whole body resulting in healthy cells being sometimes temporary damaged although they could always repair themselves. The treatment was administered using a home infusion pump which delivers the medication through a long and tin peripheral inserted central catheter also known as PICC. The infuser is made of a small hard plastic casing similar to a bottle that has an elastic balloon in which the chemotherapy drug to be infused is contained. As the balloon shrinks, the inside chemotherapy solution is pushed through the tubing connected to the PICC line into the patient's body.

PICC

This soft and flexible catheter was inserted, under sterile conditions, in a vein between the elbow crease and shoulder of my right arm. For this, a nurse in the radiology department assisted me to lie on a stretcher and used an ultrasound machine after applying a cold jelly to locate a suitable vein in the upper right arm several centimeters below the armpit. This is a conducting gel providing a clearer picture of the veins on the ultrasound screen. She also injected a small amount of local 'freezing' into the area above of the selected vein after which a needle was inserted into this part. Then, the tip of the catheter is advanced slowly through the internal vein pathways via the needle until it reaches the lower part of the superior vena cava, the largest body vein ensuring the returning of blood to the heart (Ottawa Hospital Cancer Center, 2010). It is believed that because of the large quantity of blood constantly flowing through this area, the chemotherapy medication is rapidly diluted and transported into the body. At the end, the needle was removed from the arm leaving behind the catheter. A chest X-ray was done post PICC insertion to ascertain it was in the right place and a short and clear plastic tubing to serve for the medication infusion attached to the outside part of the PICC. Then, a bandage was applied over the PICC insertion site for protection and to avoid possible bleeding following the procedure which took only a few minutes. This dressing was weekly changed and each time when the infusion of the medication was to be given. To my side, I was required to keep the PICC well secured within the dressing to prevent it from pulling out. The nurse insisted that it was very important that the PICC remained always in the same position it was initially placed as possible because any fluctuation in its length outside my body could be damaging. Some of the damage may include the folding over of the line; excessive bleeding leading to fever; pain and redness or swelling reaction at the site of insertion and in my arm, shoulder or up the side of the neck; and possible chemotherapy fluid leakage from the PICC itself.

The treatment

A 6-cycle chemotherapy regiment was prescribed and this was to be administered bi-weekly. At the beginning of each cycle, a blood sample was drawn, often from veins in both arms, for laboratory analysis at least 48 hours prior to the date of the treatment infusion. The blood analysis is done because the Oncologist wants to ensure that the level of blood counts (red and white cells and platelets) and the amount of hemoglobin and its content especially the creatinine are consistent with the required profile considering that chemotherapy causes tremendous fatigue, weakness and severe side effects. After examining the blood test results, the Oncologist could then order the amount and appropriate dose of chemotherapy medicine one should receive. Sometimes however, results from the analysis are either below or within the required limits for white blood cells. In such cases, the test was often repeated the same day, delaying the treatment administration.

When this was the case, I was always forced to wait in the room some days for about 2 hours for the Oncologist to receive, check again the test results and order the most suitable medication. It also happened some days that I had complications with the development of high fever and the drop in hemoglobin level ending up at the emergency department for medical attention and to receive additional units of blood transfusing. In such circumstances the chemotherapy treatment was momentarily interrupted until I recovered and was feeling better.

On the day when the treatment was scheduled to start, I registered at chemotherapy center, always escorted by my spouse. I introduced myself to the front desk where my file was pulled out and all necessary information recorded. Then, a nurse took me to the lounge where the infusion will take place and showed me the bed I will lie on for the infusion (Fig. 12).

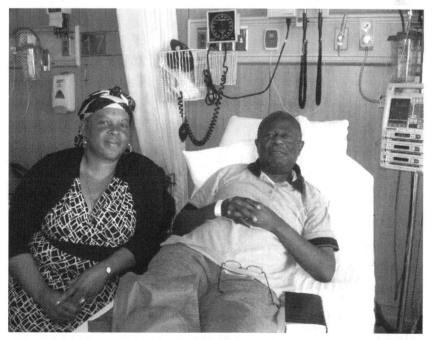

Figure 12. Lying on the bed at the Ottawa General Hospital and waiting for the administration of the first cycle of chemotherapy treatment

She then prepared all the necessary equipment including the blood pressure monitor and a computerized pump for infusion of the pre-chemotherapy medicines and fluids that help in the prevention of nausea or any allergic-like reaction as well as improve the medication delivery efficiency.

She first checked my vital signs including the blood pressure, pulse, heart rate, and respiration to ensure they were stable. Thereafter, she gave the pre-chemotherapy medications using the PICC line. Often, this process took up about 2 or 2 and half hours with each medicine having the exact time which is always signaled by an alarm from the pumping machine. At the end, the nurse double-checked my name, age and address on the medication package as well as the medicine name and its dosage (in my case it was between 3,800 and 4,000 mg) before starting the treatment infusion process. Finally, the nurse connected the infusor to the intravenous PICC and opened up the flow restrictor located at the end of the tubing to allow for a free passage of the medicine through the PICC into my body for the following days. At the end of the session, another nurse checked again the connection that has been made, and if this was done appropriately, approved it by appending his or her signature on the delivery document after which I had to leave and go home. Each treatment cycle was lasting for a 7-days period when the balloon is empty after which I had another 7-days resting time before the next connection.

Because of their harmful effects and potential accidental exposure to chemotherapy drugs by other members of my family while at home, training was also provided to ensure necessary precautions were taken during and after the treatment administration. Of particular attention was the management of my bodily waste—urine, stool and vomit which have become dangerous during treatment—to be managed properly and carefully. All the chemotherapy tools, empty infusors and tubing, and flashing needles, syringes and used gloves were always disposed of in appropriate containers. Each time I used the toilet, I always ensured it was flashed at least twice to thoroughly rinse the waste and splashes from the water flushing. Then, I had to thoroughly wash my hands with soap and rinse them well before sweeping with a towel that was designated only for my use.

Pump disconnection and treatment for side effects

When the balloon containing the chemotherapy medication became shrunk, a sign that it was now empty and the current cycle was over often after 46 hours of infusion, the home care nurse disconnected the bottle from the PICC line, wiped out the tube openings with pre-pad saturated with 70% isopropyl alcohol, flushed the line using sterile needles and syringes containing 10 mL normal saline solution, and securely tightened the PICC end with CareFusion locks. Unused syringes, needles and empty infusors were disposed in special 3.8 L chemo containers that I always then took to the local pharmacy for disposal. At this point, I had to rest and report again to the hospital for the next cycle after two weeks. Truly as time passed by, it was becoming very difficult and not easy to support the medication considering its various side effects. But, I had to bear with these regardless of the body discomfort.

They are many kinds of chemotherapy side effects but those I personally suffered from the most included nausea and some vomiting; a bit loss of appetite due mostly to dry mouth and sore making almost all the foods that were served to be tasteless than usual; partial hair loss becoming thinned; body itching mainly in the eyes which became too dry; skin rash over my extremities, trunk and face; tingling of hand palms and feet soles; loss of sensation to touch particularly when it was cold; skin burning becoming darkish in color mainly on the face and the arm around the place where the PICC line was inserted; general fatigue often feeling very tired and weak to handle any non-heavy duty such as wiping the kitchen; and numbness in feet as a result of the damage to some nerves mostly the sensory nerves as the treatment travel throughout the body to target and kill cancer cells. The later has persisted for a very long time and my Oncologist indicated that it could even take several years before it recedes. Vitamin B-12, constant massage and protection of feet by wearing good socks were prescribed as preventive measures to relieve from the symptoms. All these effects considerably interfered with my daily activities like typing on my computer, buttoning shirts and closing my belt, walking to exercise or to go to the toilet, picking items up and performing some house duties. Because my body could not tolerate any cold, precautionary measures were given by the hospital to mitigate cold effects. They were wearing always protective clothes when I had to go outdoor during cold weather, avoiding being in close contact with air conditioners or freezers and washing hands with cold water, drinking warm water and hot tea, and never taking cold foods. Special glove types were provided for use each time I open the fridge to take something.

While on radiation and chemotherapy treatments, I also became very ill with high fever but without an abnormal low number of neutrophils in the white blood cells also known as neutropenia that intervene in the primary defense against infectious diseases and drop in my hemoglobin resulting in a complete body fatigue. As a result, the treatment was temporarily suspended for a day when I was urgently rushed to the emergency department for examination of the front and lateral sides of the chest and to receive transfusion of additional four units of blood. I also underwent through other numerous physical, radiological and laboratory tests. The results of these showed that my lungs were clear with no airspace and the thorax was intact. Physical examinations by the radiation oncologist revealed I was not in distress and that there was no palpable swelling of the lymph nodes around the head or neck, no abdominal abnormal enlargement of any organ also known as abdominal cavity organomegaly and no palpable abdominal masses. In general, there was a considerable swelling at some lower extremity of my body and lack of abdominal tenderness. However, the chest was very clear and the heart sound normal. The consultation with the chemotherapy oncologist concerned mainly the drug to be given to me. He suggested that he was feeling comfortable that a

12-cycle of the medication FOLFOX should be my treatment after the surgery. He also explained to my spouse and I all the benefits, toxicities and logistics of the FOLFOX treatment. Moreover, he clearly outlined its potential risks particularly its life-threatening toxicity.

Under anesthesia, I was sterilely prepped and draped in a position lying on my back with knees bent and thighs apart which is known as the lithotomy position for an endoscopy test. Then, the radiologist inserted a flexible cystoscope through the anus into my bladder and an injection done in the prostatic urethra to raise the mucosa or blanching that is consistent with the previous radiation treatment. He successfully managed to enter the bladder without difficulty although there was a significant protrusion from the posterior to the anterior sites of the tumor. Observations indicated that there was no evidence of mucosa change—the moist tissue lining in certain parts of the inside of my urinary and digestive tracts, the trigone—a smooth triangular region of the internal urinary bladder—was normal and that there was a small flat prostate with obvious rectal tumor above it. Results further suggested that it was likely that the right ureter will need to be resected as well and probably also reimplanted. The radiologist also observed from the findings the possibility of removing the tips of seminal vesicles through the radical salvage of the tumor or cystectomy although he felt such procedure would only depend upon intra-operative findings. If such case is reached, he concluded, I will have to require anything from the ureter to complete the radical surgical treatment. By so doing, the operation will lead to removal of all organs from my pelvic cavity or pelvic exenteration with the urinary diversion via the creation of a small urine reservoir under the abdominal wall from a segment of a bowel or the ileal conduit.

Extension of sick leave

As more days went by for my cancer treatment, the Dean of the School of Natural Resources at the University in Zambia where I work called to advise that medical doctors attending to my sickness need to write on my behalf a short medical report stating the progress made and what is remaining out of the various treatments they had recommended. I discussed this with my Oncologist and he agreed to write a letter to the University on my behalf. He wrote:

June 22, 2011
TO WHOM IT MAY CONCERN:

Mr. Muimba Kankolongo is a 59-year-old gentleman with locally advanced and regionally metastatic cancer of the rectum. He is currently under treatment at the Cancer Clinic here and will be under treatment under my care for approximately 5 weeks starting in about 2 weeks' time. After this, he will have a period of 6-8 weeks for recovery followed by surgery where there will be a further period for surgical recovery. I do not know whether he will be getting chemotherapy after the surgical procedure and I do not know how long this gentleman will be required to recover after the surgery but I would expect that at the very minimum he will require at least 6 months for convalescence. Yours sincerely, the Oncologist.
THIS DOCUMENT HAS BEEN DICTATED BUT NOT READ.

Some weeks later after I had sent the oncologist's letter to Zambia which was well received and reviewed, the Dean of the School of Natural Resources at the Copperbelt University considered it necessary to apply to the University Management, on my behalf, for an extension of sick leave. In this way, I will stay officially for medical attention in Canada. The application was approved without difficulty and the extension granted. This went from 15 to 30 days first and then to 6 months which would now expire, at this time, on 31st December 2011. I become aware of this change when I received from the University Registrar Office a letter indicating the following.

The Registrar wrote:

July 18, 2011
Dear Dr. Kankolongo,

RE: SICK LEAVE

Reference is made to the letter from your medical Doctor dated 22 June 2011 in which he recommended six (6) months leave to cater for your convalescence and our letter of 14th June 2011 in which your medical leave was extended up to 30th June 2011. The Dean, School of Natural Resources has on your behalf applied for an extension of your leave and I am glad to inform you that you have been granted Six (6) months sick leave up to 31st December 2011. We hope during that period you will respond positively to the treatment. We look forward to your recovery. Yours sincerely, ACTING REGISTRAR. Copy made available to the Vice Chancellor, Deputy Vice Chancellor and the Dean – School of Natural Resources.

CHAPTER VII

TUMOR REMOVAL

*A*t the completion of the combined chemo-radiation treatment by mid-august 2011, I was completely exhausted and considerably tired and weak. I lost about 7 kg of my weight and had bright red blood from the rectum and a severe diarrhea. Several additional tests were performed prior to the surgery to reassess my health and the

While the surgery took 9 hours than the previously planned 6 hours, I could not easily open my eyes when I was transferred to the recovery unit mainly because of a double dose of anesthesia I had received.

size and whether the tumor had extended to other organs and tissues.

Medical examinations

Some of the tests which were performed included physical and digital rectal examinations, flexible Sigmoidoscopy using a fiberoptic camera to observe inside the sigmoid colon and rectum, urological consultation for a Cystoscopy, MRI, chest X-ray and full colonoscopy to rule out the possibility of other lesions that might have been missed during the early tests especially in the right and transverse colon. The sigmoidoscopy procedure helps to detect possible inflamed tissue, abnormal growths and ulcers, and any bleeding and changes that might have taken place in bowel movements. In the other hand, the Cystoscopy examines the inside lining of both the bladder and the urethra which are the channels through which urine is carried from the bladder to outside of the body. During this later test, the urologist aseptically cleaned the genital area and draped me with a sterile sheet. Then, he inserted a freezing gel into the passage after which a lighter tube or a cystoscope was gently inserted up to the urethra into the bladder. Sterile water was pumped in to expand the bladder for the purpose of having a clear view.

Test results

The uroflow test showed an excellent peak flow of urine with about 41 mL of the amount of urine left in the bladder after urination known as postvoid residual volume. There was no evidence of obstruction. The endoscopy that involved the insertion of a flexible cystoscope into the bladder without difficulty despite significant protrusion from the tumor showed no reactive change in the moist tissues lining in the urinary tracts or mucosa and that the smooth triangular region of the internal urinary bladder or trigone was normal. However, the rectal examination revealed a very small flat prostate with the tumor over the top. A follow up endoscopy under sedation confirmed the tumor had shrunk though it was still sizable and that there was no evidence of mass lesions around the tumor. It was now about 6.1 x 4.0 cm in diameter and 2.4 cm thickness. Moreover, the chest x-ray was negative for any possible spread of the cancer from one organ or part of my body to another non-adjacent organ or part which is known as metastatic disease. The chest and lungs were clear, the bony thorax intact, the heart sound normal and the abdomen very tender. Generally, It was found that the tumor has considerably decreased in its overall size and extent from 9.8 cm previously to 5.8 cm after treatments and that the urinary bladder, prostate and the iliac vessels were not affected. But, there was still concern about the tumor involvement in the right rectal plane indicating the possibility that the bladder is still affected. The pelvic lymph nodes have also significantly decreased in size and number. Their external surface was flattened, firm, focally ulcerated and appearing brown with a raised lobulated component at the proximal aspect. Though the results were showing the adherence of the seminal vesicles and prostate to the rectum on the anterior aspect, the tumor was not seen in the fibrous tissue between the two organs. However, there was a persistent involvement of the right mesorectal fascia completely surrounding the mesorectum that contains fatty tissue or mesorectal fat with a mild extension of the tumor through the upper boundary of the rectum. The performed rigid sigmoidoscopy demonstrated a good anal muscular tone or sphincter tone with no involvement in the cancer contamination of this muscle.

Based on all the above observations, it was concluded at this point to have a surgery with assistance from the urologist. In a similar endoscopy test, I was placed on a heart rate, blood pressure and oxygen monitor. Anal and rectal examinations were performed and they were normal. A scope was then inserted into the anus and passed up to the tumor which was in the mid upper rectum. Passage by the tumor and to the colostomy was without difficulty. Although the tumor had shrunk, it was still sizable but with no presence of fleshy growths (polyps) occurring on the lining of the colon or the rectum. The scope was removed after which I was placed lying on my back. The colostomy appliance was removed and the exploration of both the afferent and efferent limp was made by tracing the proximal limb from its entrance to the beginning of my large intestine or cecum which was identified by the presence of the ileocecal valve—a papillose structure having a sphincter muscle well situated at the junction between the small intestine (ileum) and the large intestine— and the appendiceal orifice that shows a complete traversal of the colon. The valve was not affected and the terminal ileum was normal. Similarly, there was no evidence of polyps or mass lesions. The scope was then carefully withdrawn and I tolerated well the procedure.

Following the pathological analysis of the rectum, the right ureter and the bilateral vesicles, it was found that the rectum had numerous foci of residual cancerous cells surrounded by a dense growth of fibrous or connective tissue. Additionally, there were a chronic inflammation and abundant foamy tissue cells such as histiocytes that are important in one's immune system as well as multinucleated giant and necrotic cells, and mineral calcium deposits throughout some of my glands known as microcalcifications. The prostate and seminal vesicles were adherent to the tumor by a fibrous tissue, but no tumor cells were seen in the fibrous tissue between the two organs. It has invaded through the region of some muscles in many organs adjacent to the submucosa membrane or muscularis propria into tissues around the colon and rectum, occupying nearly 50% of total circumference of the colon.

After discussing with the surgeon about some details on the concerns she had regarding the reanastomosis operation which is the surgical reconnection usually reversing a prior surgery to anatomically disconnect two hollow organs or anastomosis usually to restore continuity after resection and the potential for anastomosis leak after the joining together as well as various other potential complications and benefits of the procedure such as the risks that might result from changes to the bowel and bladder functions, impotence and erectile dysfunction, infection, bleeding and others inherent to all surgical procedures, I signed the informed consent form. The surgeon also clearly explained that I could end up with a permanent colostomy given the loop colostomy and the resection of prolapsed bowel I had which could have led to a very short left colon despite the mobilization of the sharp bend between the transverse and the descending colon in my left upper quadrant or the splenic flexure to bring it down and perform an anastomosis.

Though I understood well the explanations I became however so distressed about the outcome of the operation. But, the surgeon reaffirmed me there might be another window of opportunity where it might likely be that the operating team could find a way of modifying the colostomy into a loop ileostomy. If this case arises and such modifications are performed, she said, they could end up reversing it to a natural anus in future. I was so delighted about such comforting statements and I prayed for this to take place. The surgeon further discussed with me about other risks that are not related to the surgery including but not limited to the risk of wound infection, bleeding, heart attack, blood clots, pneumonia, stroke and other risks inherent with any surgery.

Surgery

By the end of September 2011, I was again brought to the operating room in a stretcher, placed on the operating table and underwent placement of an epidural on my left arm and treatments for pain management. This important surgery was to be performed by a surgeon with assistance from two other physicians among whom the anesthetist and the urologist. There were also about four nurses in the room. The procedure consisted of the resection of the low anterior and en bloc resection of bilateral vesicles, vas deferens, right ureter and portion of right posterior prostate. It also included the reimplantation of the right ureter; the taking down of the colostomy with mobilization of the splenic flexure and primary anastomosis as well as the possible diversion of the colostomy to a loop ileostomy. As earlier described, I was intubated under general anesthesia after which the operation was performed as I was asleep.

The scene, as described by the surgeon, was fascinating and far beyond my imagination. It clearly demonstrated how professional and creative the team was during the operation in which they wanted to be sure that the tumor was diligently removed together with adjacent contaminated tissues and organs. She said... "An arterial line was first placed in the right wrist. After being placed in lithotomy with the right arm tucked to the side and the left one extended, the TED stockings—stockings made of elastic fibers that are used post-surgical to squeeze legs and help promote good blood flow and prevent blood clots—were placed on the legs and an upper body warmer was used. Then, the loop colostomy was initially sutured with a pursestring and its appliance removed. After this, they washed the abdomen and then prepped and draped to allow for an adequate surgical exposure. Thereafter a catheter was placed under complete sterile conditions and intravenous antibiotics administered prior to the skin incision and then regularly redosed at 4-hour intervals. Following this, an incision was made using a skin knife from the midline cartilaginous joint between the superior rami of the left and right pubic bones anterior to the urinary bladder to just above the umbilicus. A Cautery was used to incise through the subcutaneous tissue to open up the fascia midline. They then visualize the bladder which was large and extended up along the anterior abdominal wall. It was taken down on both the right and left hand sides to have an adequate exposure. At this time, the Bookwalter was used for body wall retraction. This allowed for a complete inspection of the abdomen which revealed no evidence of the tumor spread around and through into the liver.

They then went on by taking down the distal end of the colostomy to create a window between the bowel and the mesentery and by firing a GIA-80 mm stapler after which the mesentery was divided down towards the apex, between the two limbs of the bowel. After this, the sigmoid colon was mobilized along the white line of Toldt—the reflection of posterior parietal pleura of abdomen over the mesentery of the ascending and descending colon—to enter behind the abdominal cavity or at the retroperitoneal plane. However, regardless of the presence of bulky nodes in the mesentery just near the base of the pedicle, they managed to enter the retroperitoneal plane in order to ensure a negative margin. This manoeuvre required that they took the hypogastric nerve which is located between the superior and inferior hypogastric plexus at the left side of the retroperitoneum. As they enter the indicated plane, they identified the ureter around which they placed a vessel loop before they could also observe the testicular artery or gonadal vessels and the common iliac artery located in the pelvis. From there, they then took all the retroperitoneum, the bulky nodes over the top of the common iliac artery and the interior aspect of the aorta. From the right-hand side, they scored a plane to join up to the other side. Here, the ureter was again identified in the retroperitoneum and preserved. Nevertheless, the common iliac artery was again seen and the whole tissue between the two common iliacs was removed together with the specimen.

From here, they went up and made a window above the superior mesenteric artery pedicle, which included the inferior mesenteric artery as well as a branch of the inferior mesenteric vein. There was below this a small vessel arising posterior to the abdominal aorta and superior to its bifurcation (median sacral artery) which they divided and tied with No. 2-0 Vicryl ties. The pedicle, itself, was cleared off circumferentially and then divided with scissors as well. Again, they doubly ligated my side with No. 0 Vicryl ties. At this point, they divided the remainder of the mesentery at the colon between Kelly clamps which they tied with No. 2-0 Vicryl ties. Then, they left the end-loop colostomy inside to continue with the total excision of a significant length of the bowel around the tumor. It was here that they realized unfortunately that my pelvis was extremely small and narrow making it very difficult to be dissected. In addition, they could not have good exposure because the tumor itself was quite proximal and bulky, and also due to the presence of a significant amount of fibrous tissues resulting from the radiation treatment. Despite this however, they were able to come down to the posterior plane until they could reach the curve of the large, triangular bone at the base of the spine and at the upper and back part of the pelvic cavity or the sacrum. As the plane was reached, they continued dissecting around on the left-hand side since it was like being relatively free of the tumor.

They also continued in the regular plane until they could reach the lateral aspect of the seminal vesicles. It is here that concerns arose about the proximity to the tumor. Because of this, they proceeded from the right side along the external iliac artery taking out all the tissue with the tumor including the ureter which was reflected onto the tumor surface. Then, they mobilized the bladder on both the right- and left-hand sides to identify the internal iliac vein on both sides as well as the vas deferens which carry sperm to ejaculatory ducts in anticipation of ejaculation. At this point, the urologist also intervened for the dissection. For this, they took the vas deferens on the right-hand side between ties leaving the undivided superior vesical artery inside. By doing so, they clearly exposed the external iliac, which was free, along its length although the imaging somewhat suggested that it might be at least neurologically affected due to the attachment by the tumor. Fortunately, this was not the case. However, the ureter along a very short segment – just before the entrance into the bladder – appeared to be quite fixed to the tumor. To be on a safest way to proceed with the surgery, this segment of ureter was excised down at the point it appeared to be involved with the tumor. Its distal end was tied and gently packed up into the abdomen. They went back to dissect it around the right-hand side between the seminal vesicles and the bladder. At the entrance of the bladder, they identified the ureter again and this was divided at this site in such a way that its portion was removed. The dissection continued down, keeping the seminal vesicles with the tumor on the right-hand side.

From here, they turned their attention to the left-hand side where the seminal vesicles appeared not to be clearly involved though the concern about the normal plane on the rectum. Because of this, the majority of these seminal vesicles on the left side were also taken out but the vas deferens at this side was preserved. They came through down below the seminal vesicles and the tumor by heating tissues using an electric power also known as the Bovie. While still in a plane – one layer above or anterior to the rectum – they had essentially gone below the tumor though it was still attached to the pelvic sidewall on the right-hand side and anteriorly. They then chose to continue with the dissection on the left-hand side and posteriorly going around the mesorectal plane since it was much easier on that side. In this way, they were able to come up below the seminal vesicles through the endopelvic fascia covering the anterior extraperitoneal rectum which lie between the prostate and the rectum also called the Denonvillier's fascia to get back into the usual plane. However, because of thickening on the right-hand side, they used the ligature to come through the posterior right aspect of the prostate. Once this was down, they were clearly below the tumor and again able to slowly reach back through the Denonvillier's fascia and on to the inferior aspect of the rectum. They then mobilized posteriorly again but, they soon realized that the rectum was itself very stuck to the anterior aspect of the sacrum. This encloses the sacral vessels and nerves through anteriorly to the pelvic parietal fascia and the entire pelvic cavity known as the Waldeyer fascia. They got it off the pelvic floor using tissue heating with electrical current and went around the right-hand side below the tumor to re-enter the normal mesorectal plane leading to the sidewall away. Again they realized that the pelvis was very narrow making the dissection challenging. Fortunately, they had an adequate margin below the tumor which could be clearly palpated being completely free and up. While they were still, at this point, below the seminal vesicles and on the back of the prostate, they divided the mesorectum in multiple bites using the LigaSure™ technology and a pinch-burn technique. Then, the rectum became quite visible in its full size and thickness as they had successfully cleared all the surrounding tissue and fat. A thick tissue 45 mm TA stapler was then used and fired across the rectum at this site where a sample specimen from the divided rectum was collected using a No. 15 blade scalpel for inspection on the back table. It appeared to have a complete mesorectum with a good mesorectal cuff, in line with the rectum profile. However, it was as initially suspected, quite large and thicker with a fresh minimal margin measuring about 4 cm. Its grossly negative circumferential radial margin appeared to be negative without concern of any area being infiltrated by the tumor. The rectum specimen together with the tumor (Fig. 13) was kept in formalin and sent for additional pathological analysis.

The pelvis was then re-inspected to ensure an effective control a few small areas of bleeding which had been previously managed with sutures on the back of the prostate and the pelvic sidewall. Similarly, they contained another small amount of bleeding posteriorly, previously encountered during the posterior dissection. Overall, I lost approximately 1 L of blood on the course of the dissection. The pelvis was then packed after which the surgery team's attention turned towards the creation of a colon joint or anastomosis. Since the left colon appeared it would come down in a tension-free anastomosis with mobilization of flexure, the colostomy was taken down using a knife to make a circular incision around its loop opening and Cautesy to incise circumferentially to free it also circumferentially. Once this was brought into the abdominal cavity, they easily mobilized the splenic flexure which provided even a better mobility and a tension-free anastomosis. The distal small end-loop segment was divided off and a pursestring applier and its needle were used to clamp the tissue and penetrate the tissue through the stainless-steal instrument holes across the distal end of the left colon. Then, a No. 1 Prolene suture was placed through the pursestring applier and the end of colon was removed with the heavy curved scissors. Following this, the anvil of the staple was placed in the lumen, the suture tightly tied and the anastomosis line thoroughly inspected to ensure no major blood vessels are incorporated into the staple line. They also re-inspected the retroperitoneum in the pelvis and found that the hemostasis was adequate, showing it was in its appropriate status to regulate its internal conditions so as to stabilize its health and regulate perfectly its physiological

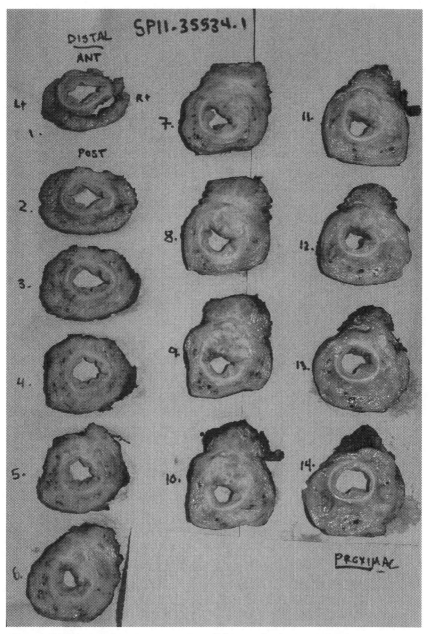

Figure 13. Fixed microscopic slides of the excised unopened mesorectum with the cancerous tumor after a 9-hour surgery

processes and functions regardless of the external fluctuating conditions. An EEA 28 mm staple handle was then placed through the anus up to the staple line after which the spike was opened and exited just posterior to the line. The staple was then placed together, closed and fired. It was later opened and removed when they found there were two intact donuts. Because of this, they performed an air test with water in the pelvis to ascertain there was no air leak, which was the case. Since there was also no evidence of problems with hemostasis, a skin rejuvenation product called Vitene was placed down in the pelvis. It was at this point that the team decided that I benefit from diversion considering the complexity of my illness and the extent of the resulting radiation changes.

I surely tell you this is a divine intervention from above. I was deeply asleep and did not discuss the idea with the surgeon prior to the surgery. Truly by His compassion and love, Jehovah who heals did not want to see his child struggles the rest of life with an external push on the abdomen through which stool eventually finds its way out of the body. Rather, His spirit descended from heaven into the operating room for the restoration of my full anatomy as I was created. Amen!

Due to the quite mobility of the terminal ileum, which easily came out through the left lower quadrant opening, they decided to use this opening to create the loop ileostomy although this has not been a standard surgical procedure. For this, they placed a single No. 1 Maxon figure-of-eight suture in the superior aspect of the opening to make it smaller. Thereafter, the small bowel was brought through the opening by creating a window between the small-bowel mesentery using a red rubber catheter to bring it up without any tension. This location was about 15 cm proximal to the ileocecal valve being the papillose structure with physiological sphincter muscle situated at the junction of the small and large intestines. The ileostomy was finally opened in its inferior aspect after ensuring for its correct orientation and brooking or grafting its superior aspect with three brooking sutures placed at 3, 6 and

9 o'clock positions, respectively. The remainder of the left-sided and diverted ileostomy was directly sutured to the skin and a rod placed at the site of the red rubber catheter....."

Stent implanting

After the tumor was removed and as I was still under anesthetic condition, the urologist in consultation with the surgeon found it necessary to insert a ureteric stent (Fig. 14) between the right ureter and the bladder to provide for a provisional channel to restore the correct flow of the urine to the bladder and allow the kidneys to drain normally. For a healthy person, usually urine formed in the kidney is normally carried to the bladder through a narrow muscular tube known as a ureter. The bladder is the reservoir where the urine is collected and when it is full, it is emptied through the urethra which is the passage to the outside the body. Due the tumor development from the colorectal cancer I was diagnosed with, a partial obstruction of the ureter was inflicted leading to only a small quantity of urine being discharged when urinating. This caused a malfunctioning of the kidneys as a result of accumulation of the urine and some infection of the urinary system often culminating to severe abdominal pain and discomfort. A stent is a tin soft hollow and flexible piece of silicone rubber tube—about 26 cm long, 1.5-6 mm diameter nearly the size of a spaghetti piece and with a curl at each end to help hold it in place—which has to be inserted in the ureter and the bladder. One curled end sits up in the kidney and the lower curled end sits in the bladder so that it does not slide out of the ureter but holding it open at the connection in the bladder.

During the surgery, the lower end of the right ureter was removed along with the tumor in order to facilitate a negative margin. The right seminal vesicle was also resected and left onto the tumor. Similarly, a substantial portion of the right side of the prostate was also removed inferiorly to facilitate a good margin as well. The remaining shortened right ureter needed therefore to

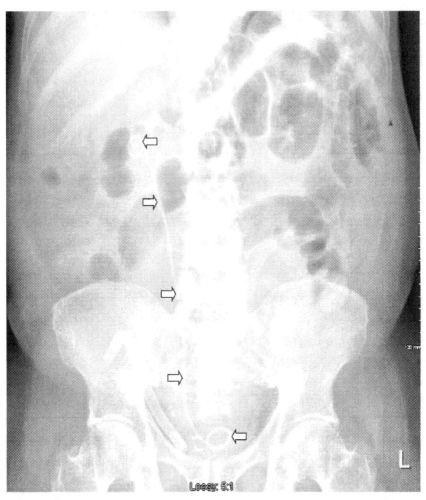

Figure 14. A stent made of a soft piece of silicone rubber of about 26 cm long and with a curl at each end to help hold in place is inserted in the right ureter between the kidney and the bladder to allow urine flow

be inserted into the bladder to drain urine from the right kidney. However, some scar tissue has developed around the area where this ureter is stitched into the bladder narrowing the opening. By inserting a stent, this section is kept open to allow the kidney drain into the bladder.

"He performed an anastomosis between the ureter and the bladder by slipping a small scope up in the pelvis— using a cystoscope for a standard technique with a running anastomosis—through the penis and the urine channel into the bladder. The right ureter was reimplanted into the bladder by passing a cystoscope through the urethra into the bladder and placing the stent in the ureter and kidney via the opening of the ureter into the bladder. The procedure—which was performed over a stent—was completed without any tension. Once the Jackson-Pratt drain was in place, the cystoscope was removed and a postoperative urine flow monitored to ensure the stent was not dislodged or obstructed. At the end of the procedure, the incision was closed with a No. 1 Maxon in a running fashion and the skin with staples. Finally, an x-ray was taken showing negative for any instruments left in the abdomen." The surgery took 9 hours instead of the initial planned 6 hours. An appointment was given to meet with the urologist 6 months after the stent placement to remove and exchange it with a new one.

In Post-Anesthetic Unit and ward rooms

After the operation, I was brought to the post-anesthetic care unit room in stable conditions according to the surgeon. She then informed my spouse, who has been in the waiting room for nearly 9 hours, that the surgery has successfully been completed and the patient is in the recovery room where he could be seen only after 2 hours. Before going back to the waiting room she obtained information about the room which has been allocated to me in the 7th floor ward and that he will be transferred over there immediately after the recovery process is completed.

She went to wait for me at the indicated room. After two hours, she realized I was not brought there and most offices were or have been closed at this late time. Then, she went mistakenly to the intensive care unit rather than the recovery room to ask why I was not transferred to my ward room up to that time. She asked about me to a staff member she met. He is not here, she said after checking for my name in her computer. Where is he then? My spouse asked again. Sorry I cannot help, she replied, adding also that you can try with the post-anesthetic care unit.

She rushed there and it was already after 6h00 pm. A nurse she met said I was still in the recovery room and she could only see me after another 1 hour. She became anxious, fearful and concerned on what was wrong that she was not allowed to see me after that very long surgery. This time, she decided to wait by the door side and after one hour, she was called to enter the room and see me but only for few minutes. The nurse asked her to follow up to the bed where I was. When they arrived, the nurse asked her to get closer to the bed to establish whether I was able to recognize my spouse. I only knew from her voice that she was by my bedside as I barely open my eyes.

"How are you?" She asked.

"Fine," I replied.

Apparently, my face was abnormally swollen. Ten minutes later which was already around 8h00 pm, she was requested to leave the room and told I will remain there for further observation because of a slow recovery of my vital signs and conscience. She left and drove home completely exhausted as she did not have either breakfast or lunch that day. I remained in the recovery room overnight, but was transferred to another ward room in the 7th floor the following day. I was now fully conscientious of where I was and what was happening around me.

CHAPTER VIII

SURGICAL WOUND AND FINAL TREATMENTS

Days after the surgery, the wound was constantly infected taking about 6 months to seal off. At one time, the decision was taken to connect the wound site to a BEDR-VAC pump to draw out the fluid leaking from it and pull the cells together to accelerate the healing. Instead, the pump sucked a large quantity of blood from my body nearly filling its collection bag and necessitating that I receive a transfusion of about 5 units of blood. I conceded for it to be disconnected and for the wound to be solely treated using antibiotics.

The wound

*D*uring the time I was still in the hospital, there was a considerable setback as the healing process of the surgery wound was concerned. The wound took a long time to heal due to several factors among which the most important were the localized collection of blood under the skin and in the body tissues or organs at the surgery site also known as hematoma, some kind of kidney failure, the continuous drainage of a profuse amount of mucus-like liquid from the wound and a constant internal infection.

Surgery wound infection

As a result of all these complications, I suffered from recurrent high fever and constant abdominal pain and infection of the wound (Fig. 15). Because of the wound infection, it was decided that the wound site be connected to a BEDR-VAC pump to accelerate the healing. The pump is a vacuum or suction machine attached via a tube to a sterile foam pad in the wound. It draws the contaminated fluid away from the wound, which is then collected in the pump siphon or canister, constituting a negative pressure therapy that works on the cells by pulling them together towards the wound center. This helps in the healing process as it stimulates the flow of both the cells and the blood to the area.

During this period of hospitalization, the pump was running properly by constantly sucking the mucus-like fluid from the wound. I was discharged about seven days later after a close observation by the nurse with speciality in surgery wounds. She visited me each day and sometimes twice a day to follow the daily progression of the wound healing by recording its measurement and taking pictures. Following observations that the healing process was on a normal path, the hospital decided that I should be discharged with follow-up health care services at home. Everything was going on well until about one day around 10h00 pm after nearly two weeks

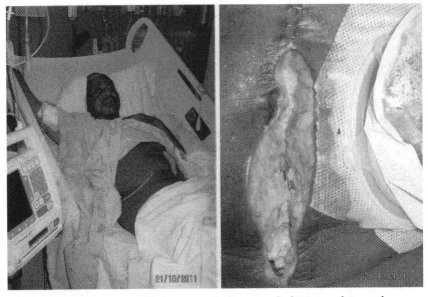

Figure 15. Infection of the surgical wound due to chemotherapy treatment that had considerably reduced my immunity system

following my discharge when the pump alarm went on making a prolonged sound. I tried to adjust it according to instructions I received from the hospital because it was full of bloody fluid, but was unsuccessful. As it continued ringing, my spouse and I agreed to call urgently back the same home care nurse who had visited me during the day to clean up the wound and change the dressings. The telephone rang for about 5 to 6 times when someone answered. As usual, the first question was to know how she could help me. I explained the problem over the telephone. Luckily enough, she said she was coming right now and hung off the telephone line. About 30-45 minutes later, someone nocked our door. My spouse went to open the door and realized she was there as promised. She rushed to my room upstairs and rapidly checked for the pump. Her only quick reaction I could remember was the exclamation..."Oh my God in the heaven..." due to the fact that the pump was full of blood rather than the leaking fluid from the wound. She could not do anything but rather decided instantly to send me back to the hospital emergency department because of the profuse bleeding from the VAC pump.

My spouse called the ambulance, which arrived within 10 to 15 minutes to take me to the emergency department. After consultation by attending nurses, I was readmitted in the hospital for a total of one more weeks mainly for the loss of blood and pain control. I was first transfused with a total of 5 units of blood after which I was simultaneously treated with pain medications; antiemetics for relieve of nausea, vomiting and headache; and the antibiotic meropenem which was daily administered intravenously through the PICC line for treatment of the wound infection up to mid-December 2011. Because of the increased blood suction from the wound site by the VAC pump, it was decided to discontinue it. The nurse in the emergency room at that time could not handle the removal saying it may result in an uncontrollable copious discharge of blood. She asked assistance from other nurses and together, they managed to remove it.

Care of the surgery wound

From this time onwards, care of the wound was well taken up using a simple cleaning of the surrounding area with alcohol prep pads, an additional wiping of the same area with 0.9% sterile saline solution, and covering it with 10.2 cm x 10.2 cm—8 ply sterile gauze sponges and tegaderm films. Though the wound was regularly cleaned and injection of a strong antibiotic provided, there was still no improvement in its healing at this time and the ensuing pain became more and more acute. Following additional instructions from resident doctors, the nurse injected me with the newly prescribed pain relief drug which, unfortunately, caused on me a bodily harm as a result of over dosage. I suddenly began to profusely sweat and abruptly, my face started to turn darkish. I began to cry loudly and relentlessly because of severe pain prompting the nurse to call urgently the surgeon.

Surprisingly that Sunday, the surgeon arrived in my room. She came hoping to observe for any improvement. Unfortunately, none was obvious. She just found me crying and slightly rolling over the bed for I was really in severe pain. My spouse asked her:

"Do you work even on Sunday doctor?"
"No," she said. She also added that
"She has just come to assess what
was going on with the patient
considering that recommendations
she has made were not applied
to control the wound and pain."

Following her visit that day I was taken for MRI tests to determine the source of the severe pain I was enduring. Results indicated that there was a failure of the kidney that was leading to an unimpeded flow of urine from it to the bladder. A small tube from a catheter was inserted in my genital organ to facilitate the urine drainage, hence decreasing the discomfort. Shortly after the tube insertion, I released urine in two urinary containers which were completely full.

I was then given an impatient room again in the 7th floor for further observations. Adjustment to medications was rapidly also made leading to a slight improvement for the wound healing as well as its sanitary appearance (Fig. 16). However, an idea rapidly came out from the attending nurse that the VAC pump should be put back on the wound. My spouse strongly supported this idea. For me, the idea of reapplying this vacuum-assisted therapy system onto the wound was over having in mind the numerous complications it had previously caused. Because of these numerous complications, the catheter was to be removed and replaced with the nephrostomy tubing by surgically implanting it by the radiologist through my skin to the right back side into the

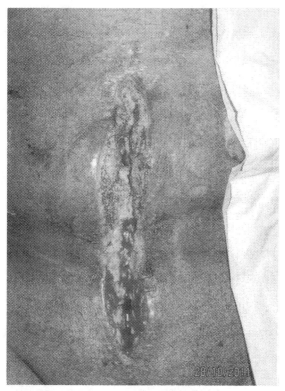

Figure 16. Improvement of the sanitary appearance of the surgical wound following infusion of antibiotics

kidney. This was done as I was continuously suffering from the ureter failure to carry the urine to the bladder. This implant was urgently to be done to avoid the kidney damage as a result of urine backing up and accumulating into it which could cause further infection. The urine was then drained from the nephrostomy into an external bag attached outside about my knee of the right leg.

Following this observation, the medical team in the urology department attempted unsuccessfully to reinsert the right-sided ureteric stent but instead, I was admitted in the hospital for a right-sided nephrostomy tube placement. During this procedure, a tube was placed through the skin on my right backside through the area of the kidney that collects urine. Once it was in place, a retrograde pyelogram was performed. This is a radiological procedure visualizing for any abnormalities of the urinary system, including the kidney, ureters and the bladder. It revealed a circumscribed narrowing of the distal ureter. Radiologists were, however, able to advance an antegrade stent down into the bladder leaving in place the nephrostomy tube. On the date I was supposed to be discharged from the hospital, they decided to pull it out under fluoroscopy but, unfortunately, it was noted that there was still an encapsulated collection of urine or urinoma surrounded by fibrous tissues—around the kidney area. A follow up nephrostogram by injecting a contrast medium through the indwelling nephrostomy catheter showed a satisfactory positioning of the double J stent and the ratio of gas in the pelvis system and the bladder or opacification, and that of the urinoma which had been previously observed. The conclusion was reached not to remove the catheter at this time. Because of this, the team decided to insert rather a more permanent nephrostomy tube prior to discharge to divert the flow from the urinoma in an attempt to facilitate the healing of the stent's orifice.

I was taken to the radiology department on a stretcher. I changed to a gown that attending nurses provided and stayed for few minutes on the waiting place before I was called. I went in the room where I was told to lay on the bed. This was too small. The nurse and the technician present in the room asked me to adjust on the bed. As I try to move the other side, I felt to the floor in pain. They rushed and pulled me up. They were worrying whether I have fractures of my head or any of my arms, legs or ribs. I said I was fine. They asked again if I was alright to ensure I had not sustained any fracture. I confirmed that I was fine. It is then they proceeded with the preparation to make me ready for the procedure. I am not sure whether the radiologist was informed about what had happened. When everything was set, the radiologist was called in to insert the nephrostomy tube which remained in place together with the stent for about three weeks following my discharge from the hospital.

The insertion was done using an ultrasound and a computed tomography to guide the needle that is first introduced into the kidney ensuring its correct position. Then a fine guide wire follows the needle through which the catheter, of about the same size in diameter as the tubing, is inserted through the guide wire to its location into the kidney. Thereafter, the catheter is connected to the bag outside the body which is used to collect urine. At this time I was connected with three different tubing devices including the PICC line, the stent and the nephrostomy beside the dressed unhealed wound. I became hampered in movement all along especially that the drainage bag had to be empty and kept below the level of the bladder all the times. It was also very difficult to sleep but with assistance from nurses, they always hang the nephrostomy bag on the bed frame at the side which allowed for a rapid movement out of the bed to reach the toilet. After finishing with the toilet use, I slowly returned in the bed and hanged again the bag at a right place where it can be reached easily. Unfortunately while in the toilet for sometimes, I realized that profuse internal bleedings resumed through the nephrostomy tube into the bag. This prompted my urgent calling of the urologist office for necessary action. It was suggested that I urgently see him at his office at the Civic Hospital. We arranged for my spouse to drive me rapidly at the hospital the following morning. After seeing the quantity of blood that was in the bag, he recommended that the nephrostomy be removed and this was done towards the end of November 2011 after radiologic examination to ensure that the stent was well in a proper position. Capsules of the medication Tumsulosin were given to be taken once a day for the relaxation of the muscles in the bladder and prostate so as to prevent the irregular involuntary urine leakage, also known as incontinence, often occurring at night times mainly after taking a cup of hot tea before going to bed.

While in the hospital, nurses also regularly rub swabs in the nose and around the rectum for analysis of possible infection from persistent antibiotic-resistant bacteria, namely *Methicillin Resistant Staphylococcus aureas* (MRSA) and *Vancomycin Resistant Enterococcus* (VRE) that are common in hospitals. The analysis is done to screen all admitted patients against these pathogens with the purpose of mitigating their spread to other patients. Infected patients are placed in a single consignment room as precautionary measures to restrict the spread. From laboratory tests, it was found that I was infected with one type prompting the hospital to regularly put me in consignment.

Pain and its management

I was constantly in immeasurable acute pain throughout the time I was in the hospital after surgery and for any of the postoperative treatments I received for the wound infection. For this, I was given a brief pain inventory chart that I needed to fill out for doctors to evaluate the pain level. It describes the pain and assesses its location in the body (knee, stomach, abdomen, head), its intensity (0=no pain to 10=worse pain) and the quality (providing the description such as burning, shooting, heavy, aching, stabbing, deep, exhausting, unbearable, constant and occasional). However, nurses regularly gave me and when needed the medications that were often prescribed by resident doctors for pain relief. They included such medication as the acetaminophen (Tylenol) 325 mg or the hydromorphone HCl 1 mg to take daily by mouth. Because these drugs could sustain my pain release only for few hours each time I take them, for instance about only 8 to 12 hours, I often felt recurrent abrupt pain discomforts after these hours. Due to their severity and the continuous discomfort I was enduring particularly at night times, I always cried for nurses' help. Often, this was because I could not sleep even after trying to position differently on the bed. When he or she reported to my room after I rang the bell, she always wanted to know first what the problem was. I described the pain and showed at which location of the body I was feeling uncomfortable which was always around the wound site. In such situations, pain relief medications were directly injected via the IV device to provide for a more rapid relief. Nurses also tried to show me how to use the patient controlled analgesia (PCA) form of pain relief (The Ottawa Hospital, 2012) which had its blue button and the intravenous patient control analgesia pump by my bed side. This method of pain relief was never used as I did not know how to use it. Despite I was still on antibiotic medications, I vigorously requested once again to the infectious disease department to recommend for the initiation of the last chemotherapy regiment to eradicate possible remnant affected cells and tissues in my body after the tumor was removed.

Medical tests

Nevertheless, the hospital decided to conduct more tests in order to establish really the source of the severe pain I was enduring. The radiogram of the abdomen revealed the presence of a mild luminal air and the swelling of the small intestine due to fluid accumulation. The air was through the colon to the level of the left colon colostomy causing a possible bowel obstruction. The CT scan after intravenous contrast viewing the pelvis in portal venous phase also indicated the presence of some free abdominal fluid surrounding the right lower ureter, suggesting the possibility of some urine leakage from ureteric connections. Another scan was performed for possible contrast extravasation—a leakage of the contrast material into the fatty tissue—from the ureter and the evaluation for possible urine leak by giving per rectal contrast. However, the scans of the abdomen and pelvis with or without contrast indicated no definitive evidence of ureteric or colorectal anastomotic leak but there were a clear small amount of a fluid collection in the pelvis and the rectal vesicular recess as well as an enlarging heterogeneous fluid collection in the mid-abdomen. These observations clearly suggested the presence of hematoma—leakage of blood into tissues outside the blood vessels—and also a possibly collection of infected fluid within the abdomen cavity. There was also a mild to moderate inflammatory in the colonic wall in the region of the hepatic flexure. The chest radiogram showed that the heart contour was within normal limits and no new airspace opacities. The thoracic scan with IV contrast gave no indication of suspicious pulmonary nodules to suggest a pulmonary disease, but there was the presence of an enlarging soft tissue nodule in the right prepectoral fat that the radiologist suggested to be reassessed using follow-up images. However, the surgeon found this to be of particular suspicious. Results of physical and blood laboratory examinations were good with normal white count and creatinine level, no palpable cervical abnormality above the clavicle, any abdominal masses and tenderness, and normal heart sounds and clear chest. The ileostomy was functioning well without difficulty.

Prior to the last chemotherapy treatment, other numerous postoperative tests including some similar to those already done were performed. They included the CT scan of the abdomen and pelvis after or without intravenous contrast and the voiding-cystography to rule out some internal leakage or collections considering the abdominal pain I had; radiography of the chest to check the position of the PICC line; CT scan of the abdomen and pelvis with IV contrast to check the possible presence of any abscess as well as some inflammation of the kidney and upper urinary tract resulting from bacterial infection of the bladder; a sonogram to assess for the distension of both the ureter and the renal pelvis with urine due to a possible obstruction of the ureter; ultrasound of the abdomen and pelvis to examine the urinary tract; flexible sigmoidoscopy and colonoscopy; general blood analysis and the carcinoembryonic antigen (CEA) test; CT scan of the thorax to check possible transmission of cancerous cells from their original site to one or more other sites in the body, usually through blood or lymphatic vessels; blood pressure; heart rate; weight; and general physical examinations of the abdomen, the whole body and at wound site as well as the status of the stoma and the functioning of the ileostomy.

Up to this time, I was still on antibiotics which started about mid-October 2011 and I was slowly feeling well, gaining weight and managing well the ileostomy which was in a good position and functioning appropriately. Similarly, healing of the surgery wound was progressing well and rapidly although there was still some leakage coming out of it and associated mild pain. It was not discharging any pus or has active infection as compared to the way it was previously. My chest was clear and the heart sound normal. The abdomen was soft and tender with no sign of any palpable mass. The blood pressure and heart rate were normal while its laboratory analysis revealed normal white cells count and acceptable level of creatinine. In addition, the kidney function was found to be excellent. Assessment of CT scan images showed that the fluid collection previously observed in the abdomen cavity had markedly decreased in size and that there was no any evidence of internal infection including any stranding or the air fluid levels within the hematoma itself. The infectious disease department thoroughly reviewed my laboratory information and declared that I was no longer contaminated with the bacterial pathogen. From these observations, which were about December 2011, the department then suggested that I discontinue the intake of the antibiotic treatment. It was after this that the oncologist had to select the date to initiate the last cycle of chemotherapy treatment which will also mostly depend on the progress of the wound healing. However, he was worrying about the delay of the treatment which could considerably affect its impact on the other cells or organs that have now been affected by the cancer and also delay or stop these from further spreading. Nevertheless, shortly after the long period of holydays at the end of December, I was so delighted to learn that mid-January 2012 was set as the date to start the chemotherapy treatment. My oncologist in consultation with other physicians concluded that I should be infused the treatment using a 12-cycle adjuvant FOLFOX drug.

Chemotherapy treatment

I was informed that the prescribed medication is a combination of three different drugs including folinic acid (leucovorin calcium), 5-fluorouracil and oxaliplatin. It was to be administered intravenously and biweekly using 4000 mg dosage. This time, I was fully prepared and well aware of what to expect during and after all cycles of the treatment. Everything went smoothly during the initial stage but things became worse in the middle and towards the end of the treatment. Regardless of what went wrong particularly the general fatigue, I had a very good appetite eating well throughout the treatment period. In fact, I always felt I needed to have some food in my mouth. I had received enough information from the dietitian on the food to eat. Instructions were to supplement my food with other sources which are rich in iron such as green vegetables as well as several other nutritional foods like fruits particularly oranges, avocadoes, grapefruits, mangoes, pears, tomatoes, pineapples, bananas, mandarins and apples to sustain my diet and provide important nutrients necessary for body energy and building capacity. These were also always supplemented by drinking either fruit juices or Ensures and Boosts that are very rich in different proteins and vitamins. I considered this as Lord's Grace when I compared myself to other cancer patients also under chemotherapy treatment.

One day, I was sitting by a lady in the hall waiting for transport after being connected to a treatment cycle. Apparently, she had a chemotherapy pump as well. I rapidly understood she was also just from the connection unit. We were both quiet as we sat there looking at different vehicles and people passing on the road through the window. Then, she bitterly complained that she cannot eat anything because of the treatment. Though she only murmured by herself, I could clearly hear what she had just said.

> What cancer have you been diagnosed with? I asked.
> She replied it was a colorectal cancer my dear.
> So do I, I quickly said.
> Do you manage to eat? She asked me.
> Yes and many times a day without any problem, I responded. She continued that she does not have appetite and she feels all the foods including water tasteless.
> I pointed out to her that she should just force eating something and try maybe 'Ensures' and 'Boosts' to help scaling up the nutrition.

Her response was that she is failing to swallow even those.

Though the husband has tried to improve them by adding some other ingredients to preventing nausea and vomiting, I am still unable to drink them. Sorry, I said. I had pity for her because she was so tin that she barely walks.

The only major problem I encountered was being unable to tolerate the cold. The last treatment took place during the pick of winter in January when the environmental weather was always below 0°C with snow everywhere. Because of this, I spent most of my time indoor going out only when I had to report for appointments at the hospital. From time to time however, I went for shopping with my spouse. In such case, I had to protect well with warm clothes. I obtained from the hospital a special type of gloves to use when opening the fridge to have water, juice or food. Instant Superex hand warmers were always also used to heat hands after using the fridge or being outside. Although I was eating well, I could not recover my full weight. The weight went from about 67-69 kg, prior to the sickness, to nearly 59 kg at that time. However, this was acceptable for me if I consider how thin I was just few months ago.

As the treatment administration progressed, I became weaker with generalized extreme body tiredness and exhaustion. But overall, I tolerated well the treatment particularly during its first course when I was experiencing only considerable numbness and tingling effects in my fingers and toes as well as some general malaise and fatigue. But, I was able to move freely. But somewhere in the middle of the treatment, it had to be momentary interrupted due to some urological issues which led to the change of the ureteric stent. The urine was not flowing smoothly again resulting in a severe lower abdominal pain. It was decided to delay the treatment considering the increased risk with the procedure of changing the stent in case I was significantly immunosuppressed at this time following the chemotherapy cycles I had already been subjected to.

While under anesthetic, the Urologist tried unsuccessfully to grasp the end of the old stent so it could be removed. It was difficult to go through the pathway due to the presence of a scar tissue that has grown over. I was then admitted in the hospital where a right nephrostomy tube was instead put in place to allow for a bypass of the stricture and get the stent down into the bladder. Using this approach, the Urologist and nurses were able to slide the old stent completely out through the nephrostomy tubing and insert the new one. During laboratory examinations, the chest showed once again some collapse of the lung that resulted in limited gas exchange or atelectasis at the right base. There was a development of some fluffy opacity associated with the atelectasis suggesting the evolving pneumonia. However, the left lung was clear and the cardiac silhouette and pulmonary vasculature normal. The PICC line and its tip were on a satisfactory position. Following the successful stent replacement, I then proceeded with the rest of the chemotherapy treatment having the nephrostomy tube in place. This went on quit well despite the side effects I mentioned early and several other issues such as bacterial infection that led to blood leakage in the nephrostomy bad.

Request for my health progress report

While I was still struggling with the above medical problems and battling in my mind over the cure from cancer about the end of January 2012, I received another call from my work supervisor at the university in Zambia requesting for the progress report on my health from any of my medical doctors. They specifically wanted to know how I was doing and when it was possible for me to get back to my work. I asked an appointment with one of my oncologists to discuss this request. I delivered and explained the message to him and he agreed to write a letter on my behalf. He wrote:

25 January 2012
TO WHOM IT MAY CONCERN:

Mr. Muimba-Kankolongo is a 60-year-old gentleman who a few months ago had a resection of his rectal cancer. He has started chemotherapy in the adjuvant setting and will continue on and off for much of the first half of this calendar year. Therefore, as his treating medical oncologist, I do not believe he will be ready to go to work until the beginning of July of this year at the earliest. If you have any further questions, please do not hesitate to call me. Yours sincerely, the Oncologist.
THIS DOCUMENT HAS BEEN DICTATED BUT NOT READ.

Surprisingly few Days later, the University responded in a way that impacted negatively and seriously on my already emotional distress I was going through. The letter I received cut my salary to half, leaving me in uncertainty as to how my rent and several other house utility bills will be paid in Zambia. My blood pressure went up sharply again increasing considerably the stress. The letter read as follow:

21st February 2012
Dear Dr. Kankolongo

RE: SICK LEAVE

Further to our letter dated 18th July 2011 granting you an extension of your sick leave, I write to inform you that following the expiry of the extension on 31st December 2011 you will now be on half salary until the time you are fit to report for work. The decision to put you on half salary is in accordance with clause 13.3.2 of your Conditions of Service. On behalf of Management I wish you well as you continue receiving medical attention. Yours sincerely, DEPUTY REGISTRAR (ESTABLISHMENT)
Copy made available to the Vice Chancellor, the Acting Deputy Vice Chancellor and the Dean – School of Natural Resources.

Night incontinence and stent change

Due to some recurrent postoperative setbacks and night incontinence, the urologist had prescribed Tumsulosin as a medication to be taken daily at bedtime for management of the leakage. He thought the problem has escalated as a result of either the stent and/or the medication. The intake was changed to morning times for few weeks. In case the incontinence was persisting, suggestions were made to discontinue completely the medication intake and then observe how it goes. Fortunately, night leakages persisted prompting the urologist to remove the stent. For this, a No. 15 French flexible cystoscope, 2% Xylocaine Jelly and standard sterile cystoscopy technique was used. Through this procedure, it was possible to observe well the urinary system. The urethra looked fine whereas the prostate was mildly enlarged. The bladder was entered and the stent had protruded from the right side of the bladder. It was grasped with the grasping forceps, removed through the tip of the penis and checked. Observations revealed that it was intact. I continued taking the Tumsulosin for additional few weeks after which it was discontinued. A further ultrasound test was performed and results showed a moderate swelling of the kidney—as a result of failure to properly collect urine—with narrowing and kinking at the insertion site of the left side, being likely the major contributing factor to the renal function decline.

A month later, the nephrostomy tube was successfully exchanged over a guidewire for an identical 10 French locking pigtail catheter under fluoroscopic guidance after injection of a small amount of contrast material into the pre-existing nephrostomy tube to confirm its satisfactory positioning within the right kidney. For this, a guide wire was inserted into the ureter under the aid of a fluoroscope—an imaging device that uses X-rays to visualize structures on a fluorescent screen. The guide wire provides a path for the placement of the stent. The new stent was then placed and advanced over the guidewire and slept it up to the kidney while watching on the real-time X-ray machine. Once the stent is in place, the guide wire and cystoscope were removed. I tolerated well the procedure and there were no acute complications. In a similar way, the chemotherapy treatment was again interrupted at this time always fearing for a potential increased risk I may face with the treatment during the time I am significantly immunosuppressed. However, the physical examination by the chemotherapy oncologist was satisfactory. He observed I was not in distress, that there were no enlargement of any lymph nodes at my head and neck areas and that the pharynx was normal with no presence of mouth sores. The chest examination revealed a good bilateral air entry with no adventitious noises. Moreover, there was no obvious sound on the heart and no pain noted upon palpation of the abdomen. In addition, there was no peripheral edema – an abnormal fluid retention – around the surgical wound. The colostomy bag was draining very well.

From the tenth cycle and almost towards the end of the FOLFOX treatment, I was feeling very bad, dizzy, nausea and feverish although I was still eating well. The chest test suggested a possible evolving pneumonia and the PICC line was still in a satisfactory position. However, I also tolerated well these conditions and forced myself for the eleventh treatment cycle. While in the chemotherapy unit where the nurse was in the process of administering initial drugs of this cycle, I vomited profusely indulging the beddings as well as the floor. I was immediately given some anti-nausea drugs and requested to stay still and relax on the bed after the sheets were replaced. I lied calmly for nearly 2 hours causing a slight delay on the treatment connection. Then after I felt a bit well, the treatment was provided and we left. On our way however, I was still feeling a general body malaise and fatigue. Suddenly again when we reached home, there reoccurred constant flowing of pinkish to reddish blood-like fluid through the nephrostomy into the bag. This was possibly the urinary tract infection again becoming a continuous problem of concern to me and my spouse. We called the Urologist who prescribed again antibiotic intake though telephone conversation. He instructed my pharmacy about the pills and the way to take them but also for further laboratory and microscopic urinalysis. In view of this continuing problem, the oncologist found it wiser not to administer the twelfth and final cycle of chemotherapy treatment as this could only cause more harm than good in terms of worsening the infection, bleeding as well as some other complications.

Though I also agreed with this plan of action, I was throughout worrying of the impact the cancellation of the last treatment might have in the killing of the cancerous cells and tissues. He requested the urologist to reassess me for the whole urinary system. As a result of my follow up visit with the urologist, an ultrasound examination was performed surveying the entire urinary system. Both the right and left kidneys were normally functioning and the stent was in a satisfactory position in the bladder performing well its functions. To absolutely ensure that the stent was in the bladder instead of previously noted pelvic fluid collection, I was given additional glasses of water and subsequently rescanned. Following this, it was confirmed that the stent was indeed in the now distended bladder and there was no drainage fluid collection in the pelvis. Therefore, the nephrostomy tube was just removed with no complications and the completion of the chemotherapy treatment became at the eleventh cycle as prescribed by the oncologist.

Wound healing

By this time, the healing of the surgery wound has progressed well with only a small scar showing on the top. I went for the collection for a blood sample to be cultured to check for any infection. After a week, results showed no signs of infection from the culture. With the continuous caring from home care nurses, they constantly checked for its healing progress when the dressings were removed to clean it. Similarly, they always scraped out the developing scar to accelerate further the healing process. They continued monitoring the wound edges and the covering scar to ensure there was no signs of any contamination such as pus, redness or swelling. In cases any of these was observed, they rapidly treated the infected and surrounding areas with an antibiotic ointment or an antiseptic powder. It was after seven full months that the wound was completely healed. However, I remained with an abdominal wall deformity – absence of the infra-umbilical abdominal wall, presence of a deep incurvation at the bottom center, scars and a hernia-like bulge (Fig. 17). Though the surgeon had initially suggested that with time the abdomen would close to reach its initial structure and restore its cosmetic appearance and physical image as the wound heals, this did not happen. I could not lose sight to my belly each time I am in front of the mirror before or after bathing. The worry that persistently came to mind was about how this deformity would affect my overall image as the abdomen contour is as much important as the other body parts in the general aesthetic structure of one's physical appearance and conditions of its peripheral skin. I constantly complained to myself about my body's image compared to its original structure prior to the surgery.

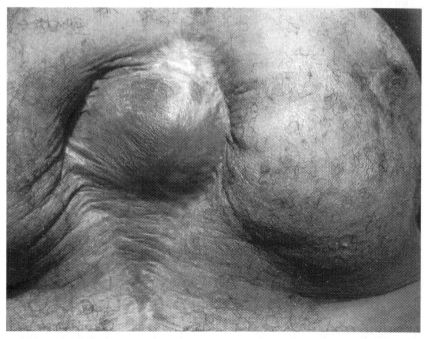

Figure 17. Wound healing 6 months after surgery leaving an abdominal wall deformity with a deep incurvation at the bottom center, a scar and a hernia-like bulge

My question to the surgeon was how this could be corrected. The surgeon emphasized that I should not worry about this deformity now as the first priority was to get rid of the tumor. Another surgery could be performed in future to reconstruct and correct the defect which has resulted from the operation for the resection of the rectum.

This operation would consist of reducing the distortion in the abdominal wall. I agreed with my doctor as all of them know what they are talking about. At this time, I was doing very well with no major complaints of pain around my incision site except some occasional discomfort on the right flank when voiding. I did not have fever, shill and weight loss and my ileostomy was perfectly functioning.

Meanwhile, the surgeon suggested that together we should now start preparing for the reversal of the ileostomy beginning with the oral administration of a Hypaque enema to prepare the colon, a flexible sigmodoscopy test, and a further assessment and management of the stent by the urologist. The Hypaque enema is enema with water-soluble radiographic contrast material. When it is administered, it produces excellent opacification of the lower and upper gastrointestinal tract and its delineation allowing an adequate gas exchange and a good observation in the bowel. I will get to the results of the treatments in due time. But first, what comes in mind was the serious problem I encountered during the hospitalization, the nursing of the surgical wound at home and the chemo-radiation treatments.

CHAPTER IX

IN THE SHADOW OF DEATH

> *I was a dead person but because of my faith in the Lord, our Healer and Savior, and my constant prayers together with those from other family members, relatives and several friends all-over the world, I was lifted from the bottom of the valley to the top of the mountain. I am healed.*

While I was hopelessly lying in various beds of the hospital wards particularly during the post-anesthetic recovery following the 9-hour surgery for the removal of the tumor, my spouse was informed that I could not regain rapidly my vital signs. Attending nurses attempted for a long time unsuccessfully to wake me up. In medical terms, this was a clear sign that I was dead. But by the grace of His Majesty, my LORD in the heaven, the monitoring system started to indicate some signs indicating the beginning of recovery and then slowly

I open eyes. It is at this time when the nurses asked her to enter in the recovery room so that they could establish whether I was able to recognize her.

One the nurses asked me....
"Do you know who is here?"
"Yes," I replied with again my eyes closed.
"Who is the person standing by your bed side?" She asked.
"My spouse," I said.
I said so because I could clearly hear her voice though my eyes were not open at that time.
Then, my spouse asked....
"How are you feeling?"
"I am good," I firmly answered regardless of some abdominal pain I was feeling.

After this question and answer interactive communication, she was given my designated inpatient room number in the ward upstairs to go there and wait for me. She waited for a very long time and realized I was still not transferred that night as the nurses wanted to follow closely my recovery progress. She left the hospital after she was informed that I will remain in the recovery unit that day. During early hours of the following day, I was transferred to my room after all the connection lines to the oxygen and water were removed. I found my spouse already in the room. She narrated how it was hard for her to locate me after the surgery as well as the stress she endured because of the long surgery. My eyes were now open and I could properly follow what she was telling me. However, I constantly felt severe pain in the abdominal area that did not allow for a comfortable rest. Often when the acute pain recurred, it triggered in me that feeling of loss of hope for everything in life. It always was so painful prompting my beliefs that I was going to die. When I was able to close eyes so as to sleep hoping my bed would comfort me and ease the pain to forget momentarily the hardship and suffering, then were a multitude of terrifying nightmares full of bad dreams and scary death visions. Often, I abruptly woke up and checked when the night will end to give rise to the day. Nights were always very long deepening the kind of groaning around the surgery wound and my weeping all along.

Dreams

Throughout the journey of my sickness, my spouse and I spiritually talked with the Lord in dreams. I stayed once in a room that I shared with another patient in his elderly age. During the afternoon of one day, he received a visit from relatives among which were two children, a boy and a girl in their younger age, and their parents. It was also apparent that his neighbors were in the group. While adults were discussing about his sickness, the children were in the contrary very busy running around and having fun. Everything was good for them probably because they were in presence of their grandfather. At times, they came to my bedside and asked what my name was. After I pronounced all my names, which they were unable to repeat easily, they ran away and then came back. What is your name again? They asked. Before I could repeat it, they were called by parents may be thinking they were disturbing me. Instead, their running around and questioning distracted me from the acute pain I was enduring. After few minutes as the room became quiet, I closed eyes and slept deeply.

In my sleep, I had a dream his visitors praying loudly at my roommate's bedside. They asked me to join them for the prayer. I agreed and left my bed to go where they were assembled. When I reached the place, I realized there were in a group including the same two children and their parents as well as the patient himself and two other ladies from the hospital management. We began to pray together loudly and at the end, one of the hospital staff asked me to kill my spouse. She was trying to give me a sharp knife she had in one hand as a weapon I should use to kill my spouse. As surprised and shocked as I became, I refused to take that knife and said it was not possible to do so because The Lord we are now praying is the same God my spouse prays too. He is the same God who protects and heals us, I continued. Because of my refusal to commit the murder she had planned, she then said she was leaving for her office and if we needed anything from her, we should meet with her in the office in room 252 of the same floor. I woke up and noticed to my surprise that about four nurses were busy transferring my roommate to another room and everyone among his visitors was standing there watching. Astonished by the move, I asked where my roommate was going. They said he has been transferred to room 252 just across the hall. I suddenly said to myself that this should be the office of the administrative officer who wanted me to kill my spouse I have just saw in the dream. I remained quiet but with considerable fear. They ended the transfer but returned to clean up the place and rearrange the bed in readiness for another patient. Few minutes later, his relatives came to pick up some of his items which were still in the room and the children were crying by saying…. "Grandfather please come back, please come back…" Because of this unfolding event I quickly asked how he was doing. The answer I got was really disturbing. Unfortunately he could not make it, they said. He just passed away few minutes ago. When my wife arrived, I related to her everything I saw in the dream and its ending. A day later, one ward manager came to inform me that another room has been found where I will be transferred and leave this one for other patients. I quickly reacted that I hope this should not be room 252. Why not that room? She asked. I just told her that it was because of the dream I had the previous day regarding that same room. I described to her everything I saw in the dream about my roommate and room 252. I now understand, she finally said. They looked for another room where I was transferred for the remaining time I spent in the hospital at that time.

My spouse and I had several dreams during that same period, all clearly pointing to an imminent death in the family.

In another stroke of a dream, my spouse saw the following while sleeping just few days later after my dream. She had come to visit me in the hospital and was standing by the window side near my bed. She realised there were a nurse with two other male persons the other side of the window but near to it. Then she asked politely. What are doing here? They replied that they want to come in after you leave. To do what my spouse asked again. They quickly responded that we have been sent by this person to kill your husband. The name they had indicated was that of one of my closest friends who is no longer with us on hearth. He passed away nearly 5 years ago due to a heart attack from the time of the dream. If that is the case, I will not leave and we shall see how you get access to the room to commit your offence my spouse retorted. Because she did not comply with their request, they just jumped on her trying to push her outside the room. She fought back aggressively and fortunately, she managed to lift and throw all of the three persons out to the other side of the window. As she tried to see whereabouts they will go, she woke up in considerable panic and sweating.

Following my wife's dream, I had another nightmare while having a nap, this time, on our bed at home about two weeks after I was discharged from the hospital. As I closed eyes, I discernibly saw the spouse to the same friend involved in the above dream trying to strangle me. She was also hardly pulling my hair. I easily recognised her face because she was on top of me firmly sitting on the area where I had the surgery wound. I could also clearly ear her saying this time you are not going to escape because I will finish with you. I fought back as she continued crushing my throat. During the fight to release myself from her hands which were around my neck, I was crying powerlessly and loudly citing her name that "please leave me, leave me alone please." My spouse who was in the room heard my talking and cry while sleeping and also realized how I was agitating on the bed and weeping with eyes overflowing with tears. She woke me up and asked what is it that you are crying while sleeping and citing this person's name. As I opened eyes, tears dropped to my face side into ears. I wiped the eyes and the face, and told her what I just saw in the dream. She prayed for me and I went back on my sleep.

In another dream few days later, my spouse had a ride in a bus full of many women passengers. When the bus arrived at the station where she had to drop, she asked where she could find the hospital to the other passengers. She was told to wait for another bus going in the other direction. Once in the bus, she can then ask to the driver who will surely indicate where she will drop and found the hospital. She waited for a while and then boarded the bus. While in the bus but nearly reaching the place she was supposed to get out, she was given the hospital direction. The hospital was just across the road. She waited for few minutes for the road to clear up before crossing to the other side of the road. Then she saw the car of one of our pastors also coming to the hospital to visit me. They were three people inside, the pastor who was driving, her spouse and their daughter. She did not stop them to enter the vehicle rather she just showed them the place where they could park the car. As they drove to the parking lot, she crossed the road to join them, and together they start coming to the main entrance of the hospital. When they enter, they realized that another pastor from a church where my spouse is a member was already in the visitors' space waiting for my spouse. After greeting each other, they said the meeting should now start. Just few minutes after they started discussing, a nurse came rapidly towards my spouse to indicate that she should rush to that room—which was my inpatient room— because someone inside was badly crying. She left the meeting and run to open the door. When she entered, she realized my arms and legs were tight together with the whole body to a chair, and someone was beating me with a baseball bat. I was crying to death and tears were profusely dropping from my eyes. When that person saw my spouse in the room, he stopped what he was doing and left angrily. I pushed painfully the chair where she was. She untightened me from it and I failed myself into her arms. She woke up.

To my side in another dream two months later, I saw that the twin cab Toyota Hilux pickup I was driving for my work has now become my coffin. I was lying on the seat of the vehicle when people were burying me. During the burial, I tried to get out but those people were saying it was too late to escape. They continued adding soil to the thumb to completely cover me. Forcibly, I woke up and realised that I was dreaming. When my spouse came for a visit, I described again the dream I had in the night. We prayed together and then concluded that there was a spirit of death rooming around me. Moreover, it is written in the scripture of Job in the Bible that (Biblical quotations in this book are taken from The Holly Bible, NIV, 1984):

> JOB 33: 14–18
> ....For God does speak– now one way, now another–
> In a dream, in a vision of the night,
> when deep sleep falls on men
> as they slumber in their beds,
> he may speak in their ears
> and terrify them with warnings,
> to turn man from wrongdoing
> and keep him from pride,
> to preserve his soul from the pit,
> his life from perishing by the sword.

Dreams are part of important tools through which the LORD shows something that may happen. I surely knew that believing in our Savior, The Lord Jesus Christ and having faith in the Majesty will instantly turn my desperate situation into a joyful one. So, thoughts came to mind that only the LORD would strengthen me, deliver my body from the suffering and keep me alive. My spouse suggested we inform some pastors about these dreams so that they advise and help to cast out the looming spirit of death.

Faith in THE LORD

All these events did not discourage my spouse and myself, and could not divert us from the faith we have for the protection and the healing power of THE LORD JESUS CHRIST for it is written: ....

"Is any one of you sick? He should call the elders of the church to pray over him and anoint him with oil in the name of the LORD. And the prayer offered in faith will make the sick person well; the LORD will raise him up. If he has sinned, he will be forgiven. Therefore confess your sins to each other and pray for each other so that you may be healed [JAMES 5: 14-16]."

He is our Lord, the Healer (Spangler, 2004) and He died on the cross for our salvation. The Holly Bible was brought to me in the hospital and starting this moment, I slept with it by my bedside all the times for I knew it is the only weapon which would save my life than Satan who will rather want to kill and destroy it.

It is also written in [JOHN 10: 9-10] that:
Jesus said..."I am the gate; whoever
enters through me will be saved.
He will come in and go out, and find pasture.
The thief comes only to steal and kill and
destroy; I have come that they may have life,
and have it to the full."

Reading the Bible and other evangelical materials

From that day onward, I committed my time to be reading regularly at least four chapters each time the Bible is open. My reading began from the New Testament and at the end, it continued with Genesis. The whole book by Job [JOB 1: 1–42: and 17] was inspiring and significantly enhanced my faith in the supernatural power of THE LORD for healing. The Bible contains several scriptures which refer to the healing and reading these God's Words made my mind up to declare healing every time rather than expecting death. Some of such important scriptures are found in:

JEREMIAH 30: 17-1 when the LORD declared:
....But I will restore you to health
and heal your wounds,...

This was the Word of God concerning the restoration of Israel. He did it then, so shall he do it again today for me for he takes away all sickness.

The Bible healing stories for the man with leprosy, that of the centurion's servant, a dead girl, a woman with a chronic blood leakage problem, and several others are clear indications of God's will for His people's health.

LUKE 5: 12-14
While Jesus was in one of the towns, a
man came along who was covered with
leprosy. When he saw Jesus, he fell with his
face to the ground and begged him, "Lord, if
you are willing, you can make me clean."
Jesus reached out his hands and touched
the man. "I am willing," he said. "Be clean! And
immediately the leprosy left him.
Then Jesus ordered him," Don't tell anyone,
but go, show yourself to the priest and offer the sacrifices
that Moses commended for your cleansing, as a testimony
to them.

MATTHEW 8: 5-13
When Jesus had entered Capernaum, a centurion

came to him, asking for help. "Lord, "he said, "my
servant lies at home paralyzed and in terrible suffering."
Jesus said to him, "I will go and heal him."
The centurion replied, "Lord, I do not deserve
To have you come under my roof. But just say the word,
And my servant will be healed. For I myself am a man
under authority, with soldiers under me. I tell this one,
Go, and he goes, and that one, Come, and he comes.
I say to my servant, Do this, and he does it.
When Jesus heard this, he was astonished and
Said to those following him, "I tell you the truth. I have
Not found anyone in Israel with such great faith....Then
Jesus said to the centurion, "Go it will be done just as you
Believe it would." And his servant was healed at that hour.

MATTHEW 9: 18-19, 23-26
While Jesus was answering questions about fasting,
A ruler came and knelt before him and said, "My
Daughter has just died. But come and put your hand
On her, and she will live." Jesus got up and went with
him, and so did his disciples....
....When Jesus entered the ruler's house and saw the flute
players and the noisy crowd, he said, "Go away. The girl
Is not dead but asleep. But they laughed at him. After the
crowd has been put outside, He went in and
took the girl by hand, and she got up. News of this spread
through all that region.

MATTHEW 8: 17
The healing power of the LORD Jesus Christ was to fulfil what
was spoken through the prophet Isaiah:

"He took up our infirmities
and carried our diseases."

In recent time however, supernatural healings of sicknesses are many to enumerate and constitute further proof that our Lord Jesus Christ is alive. If He did it yesterday, He will do it today, tomorrow and forever. Reading stories in the Bible like the above calls for an awakening and self-examination of the past, but also creates new perspectives and opportunities to enlist you into a strong faith in God.

In addition to the Bible, my spouse and family's relatives and friends provided other additional evangelical resources including books and magazines for reading. All these materials considerably assisted in the development of my faith in God who has taken upon my sickness and every pain and suffering. Of particular importance were those magazines brought by a pastor, woman of God, from Gatineau in Quebec who had been regularly visiting to console and exhort me with prayers for faith in the healing power of the LORD both in hospital and at home. It also happened that the pastor is my spouse's elder sister. They included The Word of Faith by Kenneth Hagin Ministries; Believers's Voice of Victory by Eagle Mountain International Church Inc./Kenneth Copeland Ministries Inc.; the 199 Promises of God (Babour Publishing, Inc., 2007); How to Study the Bible; You are Healed (Copeland, 1979); Healed of Cancer (Osteen, 2003); Faith Will See You Through (Pagels, 2010); From Faith To Faith: A Daily Guide To Victory (Copeland and Copeland, 1992); Woman! Thou Art Loosed (Olukoya, 2004) and Praying with Fire (Billet, 2002) to cite but a few.

In the magazines, I came across many inspiring stories that helped me in attaining greater height in my walking with my Master, the Lord Jesus Christ. I also became fond of watching some Christian television networks like the DayStar, Trinity Broadcasting Network (TBN), Grace Vision and others such as Bobby Jones Gospel at BET and Bill Gaither worship musics, and listening to radio channels like the family radio in search of God's Words. Not only these kept me busy and away from the pain I was enduring, but also reaffirmed and strengthened my commitment to Jesus Christ as my Savior, Provider and Healer. In Kenneth Hagin Ministries' 2009 *Word of Faith* magazine, I discovered the following confession—reproduced with courtesy from the Ministries—that I adapted as my daily prayer.

Prayers from men and women of God

Several pastors including men and women from different denominations and one apostle visited in the hospital and at home to pray for my healing. The hospital chaplain also visited regularly for prayers while being hospitalized. As my spouse had suggested following those death dreams, one of the local pastors was called and informed about these. He came to visit in the hospital together with his wife who was nearly at the term of her pragnency. The visit coincided with that Sunday when the surgeon passed by to check on my wound and the level of pain. In his prophetic vision, the pastor interpreted the dreams just as we had previously said. He stated that all were clearly pointing to a prominant death in our family. It also happened that I was booked for an MRI examination that day. When I was picked up in a stretcher for the MRI laboratory, they remained talking with my spouse in the room. After the test, I was again brought back on a stretcher and put back on the bed with assistance from the porter and nurses. Then the pastor immediately said "he is seeing in a vision that there is a certain woman in DR Congo sitting on a bucket full of blood and claiming that this is my blood. She is also asking why you, as a prophet, are praying to protect for his life. Do not protect him. You should get out of this place, she added."

Finaly, he requested that I close eyes and bow to pray. As he started praying deep into the spiritual realm, he suddenly engaged himself in a very dangerous prayer of trying to attack and destroy all the demoniac spirits assigned to kill me.

He said: "Almighty Father, I pray in the name of the Lord Jesus Christ of Nazareth for instant healing of the patient and curse any form of spirit of death in

Heavenly Father, thank You for being my Father. I have been born again, and I am Your child. Thank You that Your great plan of redemption includes healing for my body.

Mathew 8: 17 says that Jesus took our infirmities and bore our sicknesses. What He bore, I need not bear. It is also written, *"...by whose stripes ye were healed"* (1 Peter 2: 24). If I *was* healed, I *am* healed. I believe that in my heart and I say it with my mouth.

Because Jesus bore sickness for me, I am healed. I am free. I no longer have sickness or disease. Thank You, Father, that Your will for me is that I be well, and that I live out the full length of my life without sickness, pain or disease.

him and in this family. I cover them with the blood of Jesus Christ for the protection for no weapon that is formed against them shall prosper. I command in the Holly name of Jesus Christ, he continued, that this bad spirit leave the patient and the family and come into me now. I command that the Holly host fire consume all the agents of Satan that were assigned to attack and kill the patient and proclaim complete victory from Satan in the name of Jesus Christ. I thank you Jesus, he concluded, for the healing he has received. In your name we have so prayed, Amen."

Altogether we replied.... Amen!.

After the prayer, we stayed discussing for several hours. The conversation was mainly centered around my sickness and the progress that might have been achieved in the recovery. He ensured me not to worry about it because God has taken it in His hand and that everything will be allright. They said bye! bye! and left. It was about 6h00-7h00 pm. About 10-15 minutes after they had just left, my spouse's cell phone rang. When she took it, the prophet was on the line saying that they have just been involved in a serious car accident. Someone has hit their vehicle on the side where the wife was sitting and she has been rushed to the hospital while he left at the scene of the accident with the police investigating the cause. He provided the direction of the place where the accident took place. My spouse took her bag and rushed to the place. When she reached there, she realized this was a clear spot where any accident could not be expected. The vehicle was completely damaged and the prophet was trembling and lacking words to explain to the police how the accident had happened. After the recording of all the facts ended, my spouse took him and they went together to the Civic Hospital where his spouse was taken. A report was given that she might have her hip fractured and that the hospital was going to force the childbirth through induction of labor or caesarean section before any intervention. Through the procedure, a baby girld was delivered that day and prior to the predicted date. She was kept in an incubator in a separate room from the mother for a while.

When the mother recovered and became in stable conditions, she underwent some surgerical operations after which she could only use supporting canes to walk. However, she went through some rehabilitation processes to accelerate her walking ability for several months. Following these, she recovered and both the mother and the child are currently in good health. She does not use anymore those canes as walking support.

In about three weeks after the accident, the pastor, his spouse and the baby visited our home to follow up on the progress on my health and this was until the wife had fully recovered from the injuries. When they visited, I was still with the PICC line being used for the chemotherapy treatment and was carrying the colostomy pouch for release of stool as well. I requested for my spouse and his wife including the baby to leave us with the pastor in the sitting room. They went in the basement where we have arranged another place with a TV for visitors. As they were away, I took the occasion to confess my sins, repent and surrender myself to the LORD so that my heart will not reproach me in anyway of any wrong doing during my past. He ointed me with oil, laid his right hand on my head and prayed again for me. As he was praying, I felt something strange in my body and I abruptly felt shaking powerlessly on the floor. My eyes were closed, the body sweating and I was saying with a very faint voice "Thank you Jesus, Thank you Lord". After about 10 to 15 minutes or so prostrating myself to the ground and glorifying the Lord for the peace that suddenly came in me, I managed to stand up anyway whithout energy. My shirt was completely wet. It took at least sometimes for me to come back to normal after which we continued with our discussion. Our spouses joined us in the sitting room where we spent about an hour or so before they left. It was already in the evening time. Before leaving, the pastor said to me that I have already been healed and that I should not worry too much about the situation.

Prayers from the family and friends

My spouse continued praying always pleading to the LORD for my healing and recovery. The prayers were done wherever she was; either at home, in the vehicle, at work or also and often at her friends' places. At times, we prayed together using some books such as "Praying with Fire" by Barbara Billet (2008). In this book there is a specific prayer which is recommended when one is in need of the healing. The author has also provided numerous inspiring testimonial evidences from those who had spoken God's words based on the book. Additionally, my spouse and other women regularly have retreats each year in their Ministries during which either prayers are done based on a given request, bible studies are conducted or speakers are invited to lead discussions in any topic of interest and/or concern from the biblical point of view. It just happened that while I was in the hospital seriously sick and having considerably lost weight, they had planned for one that period. Because she was the organizer, she started battling with her mind whether she should go and attend the retreat or just make excuses to herself because the husband was very sick. While she was still questioning in her mind, God's words strongly came to her and gave instructions that she should attend. She asked me about her going for the retreat and leaving me alone in the hospital. I rapidly replied that she should travel to the retreat place and gave a request to the other members to pray for my healing. So, she left that evening to join other participants to the site of the meeting. No one knew that she has a sick person in the hospital.

It is when she gave a prayer request to the women of faith like her to pray for her husband who has just been operated and still hospitalized at the onset of the retreat that everyone was surprised. Then, all the members began praying by sending God's words in my life mainly according to the scripture as written in [Psalm 107: 20]. They prayed for the Lord (Fig. 18) to send His Words of healing to me and also asking to the Lord to give His

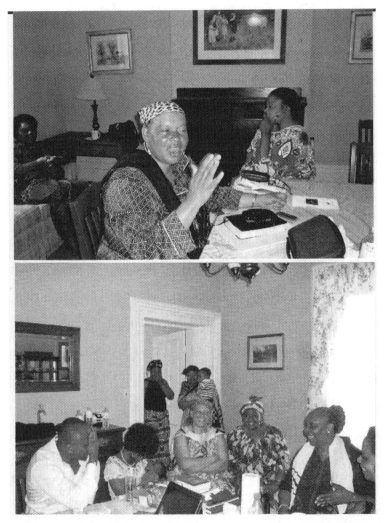

Figure 18. My spouse and her colleagues from the El Rapha Women Ministries praying for various requests including my recovery (above) and sharing the word of God (below) during the retreat in March 2012

Angels' charges over me and to keep me safer in the hospital as she was away to take care of me as written in [Psalm 91: 11]:

> "…For he will command his angels
> concerning you
> to guard you in all your ways;…"

While in the hospital and my spouse at prayer meeting, I encountered the first miracle. I felt bowel movement prompting me to rush to the toilet. I initially thought the stool will run through the colostomy. But as I stood in the toilet, I realized that it was like running through the normal anal channel. I sat and to my surprise the stool came from the anus for the first time. I thanked the Lord and rapidly informed my spouse about what I have seen.

After three days of prayers, the retreat ended and my spouse went back home to check on the kids first before coming to the hospital. To her astonishment, I was feeling well and was discharged the next day. But unfortunately, the devil said he was not finished with me yet for I became again very sick just few days after the discharge. She urgently called the ambulance to take me back to the hospital emergency department because the situation was getting worse than before. As I was re-admitted in the hospital and her sitting by my bedside, she clearly heard the devil asking the following: "Are you going to bury him if he dies?" She was shocked and suddenly became so mad to Satan in her spirit. This event prompted her to change the way in which she has been praying. Starting this moment onward, she adopted a warfare prayer according to the scripture as written in [Luke 10: 19] which says:

> "..I have given you authority to trample on snakes and scorpions, and to overcome all the power of the enemy, and nothing will harm you.."

She used this approach treading upon all the sicknesses and diseases in the family, and upon every spirit of death and hell around me. [Jeremiah 1; 10] says that:

> "..See, today I appoint you over nations and kingdoms, to uproot and tear down, to destroy and overthrow, to build and to plant."

She continued praying by using these biblical Words days and nights to root out all sicknesses, to pull down diseases and destroy every seed of cancer in my life. Moreover, she prayed to build the wall of protection around me with the blood of Jesus Christ because she knew that God's Words in [Revelation 12: 11] say that:

> "They overcome him by the blood of the Lamb and by the word of their testimony; they did not love their lives so much as to shrink from death."

as well as to build the wall of fire around me according to the scripture in [Zechariah 2: 5-7] which states that:

> "..And I myself will be a wall of fire around it, declares the LORD, 'and I will be its glory within.' Come! Come! Flee from the land of the north. "declares the LORD," for I have scattered you to the four winds of leaves," declares the LORD. 'Come, O Zion! Escape, you who lives in the Daughter of Babylon!"

After all the prayers, she planted the Lord's healing words over me. And today, she indicated that she sincerely thanked God for the power of healing over me because I am now so strong and healthy. "Praise be to the Lord" she will always shout.

In line with the retreat, another woman of God from the US was invited in 2011 and was hosted at our house before and after the meeting. After learning that I was sick with cancer, she began interceding unceasingly by pleading to the LORD for my healing during her stay and after the retreat when she returned back to the US. In the following retreat organized in 2012, another speaker also a woman of God but from another Province of Canada came to visit me at home for a short period in a company of her friend. They consoled my spouse with prayers about my sickness. They prayed for several hours for my healing after which we stayed for a while discussing about many things but mainly the Lord's Words from the Bible. We all realised that one of the topics in our discussion was interesting that it could be considered for the following year retreat. Arrangements were made that she could return and speak to the woman group about it in 2013. Unfortunately, I was again hospitalized during that period but we agreed that my spouse stay with other women at the retreat place for the three days the meeting was going to take place. During the gathering, my prayer request was considered together with those of several others. Members always agreed with my family in prayers for my healing. I salute them in the Holy name of the LORD Jesus Christ. In the similar way, other members of our family including my brothers and sisters, and consanguine relatives either in DR Congo or in other countries around the globe, and those of my spouse here in Canada and elsewhere also persistently had me in their daily prayers for my healing and quick recovery. Their pouring emails and constant telephone calls for conversation highly comforted me. We always agreed together for the Almighty's healing of my sickness. Their common persistent message that God in heaven will protect and heal me was always so encouraging.

As it was with the family members, so did other friends everywhere pray pleading to the LORD for my healing. They also constantly called or mailed letters from different countries where they reside such as Canada, Côte d'Ivoire, France, Germany, Italy, United States, Democratic Republic of Congo, Zambia, Malawi, Angola, Nigeria, Benin, United Kingdom and South Africa for their prayers of healing and to wish me for a quick recovery. Among them were some very old friends I met during childhood while others were those I met during secondary and graduate education, and still others were workmates and some I became friends during the past recent years. Surprisingly, all of them conveyed the same feeling of concern about the sickness I have been diagnosed with. Some knew it while others did not. Those who knew cancer as a dangerous disease may be fearing it for its devastating impact on human life but those who did not have any information about it, particularly those still living in rural settings of sub-Sahara Africa where I was born and spent most of my time, may just consider that one is affected by a normal sickness. Yet, cancer has become one of the death leading diseases worldwide and necessitates more expensive equipment and medications for its diagnosis and treatments. As days, weeks and months went by, they continued calling or writing throughout to get information on the progress of my health. Their warm attachment and love to me and my family remain the true reflection of God's love. They all continue caring about me.

CHAPTER X

TREATMENT RESULTS AND SURGERY

*A*fter all the treatments I went through in the General, Civic and River side Hospitals as well in other clinics including numerous medications, blood transfusion, chemotherapy and radiation regiments, and the four surgical procedures, the most important moment I have been waiting for was to know the outcome of their impacts.

After going through various treatments and surgeries, the final tests showed no sign of cancer from my body. I was declared cancer survivor with recommendations to have follow up tests each six months for the next two years and then each year for five years.

Unforgettable October 2012

My spouse and I met with the chemotherapy Oncologist on Friday 2nd October 2102 in a consultation room at the General Hospital to find out what transpired from the last examinations following the surgery to remove the tumor and the 12-cycles FOLFOX chemotherapy treatment. They were the CT scan of the abdomen and pelvis without intravenous contrast, the chest X-ray also without intravenous contrast and the CEA blood analysis. Shortly after we have been waiting, the physician entered the room and sat, holding a large folder. He asked: "how are you feeling?" "Very well doctor" I replied. Then, he opened the folder searching for about 3-5 minutes the page with the test results. My spouse and I were quietly looking at him and my temper was high. I was trembling and anxious to hear the results of the treatments. The heart and my bones were trembling, the heart beating rapidly at an abnormal rate. I felt as it has jumped out of its normal place. If the blood pressure was recorded at that time, it would have reached the highest level I ever had. When he reached on that specific place in the folder, he hit on the paper with his left hand and said five important words that I will never forget the rest of my life. He said smiling that "all the tests were excellent". My heart's beating rate, which had nearly doubled as we were waiting to hear from him, suddenly returned to normal. The screening of CT scan images, he continued, revealed improvement in the swelling of the kidney that resulted from the obstruction of the urine flow known as hydronephrosis as well as that of the postoperative formation of the excessive fibrous or scar tissues called fibrosis. He concluded that the most important observations were that the CEA was perfect and there was no sign of cancer in the body any more. On behalf of the entire medical doctors who were involved in my case, he declared me a new cancer survivor. He also made several follow up recommendations that I will have to stick to. I cried with joy after hearing those good results and glorified The LORD for the healing. I said thank you to him and to other physicians, though they were not with him in the room, for their great effort and willingness to save my life.

Follow-up recommendations

The oncologist stated that while I have now been released from the hospital regarding the treatments of your sickness, I refer you for post-treatment follow-ups to your family physician for the following next five years. In addition, he said, I will need to do the scanning of the body again within the first 6-month period after the current tests and thereafter each succeeding year for the next 5 years. Eat well particularly vegetables and fruits, and exercise regularly, he added, mainly because a good diet and being active constitute one of several factors that are not conducive for cancer recurrence and development. According to the American Institute for Cancer Research (http://www.aicr.org/foods-that-fight-cancer/), a diet which combines a variety of plant foods such as vegetables, fruits, whole grains and beans, and limits red meat and avoids processed meat highly helps in lowering the risk for several cancers. Moreover, it has clearly been shown that physical activities will have considerable positive impact on the body vigor and vitality; cardiac respiratory fitness; possible depression and anxiety; and potential weight gain during the adulthood. The Oncologist also emphasised on my strict avoidance of smoking and excessive alcohol intake in case I were obsessed of these. Further, he requested that I contact the Ottawa Regional Cancer Foundation for a 1-month training program on cancer survivorship care known as Wellness Beyond Cancer Program. The Program provides support and guidance once cancer treatment is completed. Finally, he concluded that they were pleased of my recovery and the progress I have made to keep up with a good health life. He pointed out that I was looking very much in good health now compared to the very day I was first admitted to the hospital. I replied that I was also so glad of the outcome and will follow step by step as advised in my outpatient plan on living well and managing the health after cancer.

Prior to meeting with the chemotherapy Oncologist who has just discharged me from the hospital, I had a checkup with the radiation Oncologist. Physical examinations revealed I had no distress as well as no any palpable enlargement of lymph nodes around the neck and the clavicle. Moreover, he indicated that there was no sign of cervical or supraclavicular adenopathy. The internal noise test revealed that my chest was clear and that the heart sound was normal despite the presence of a faint whooshing murmur. There was neither any palpable abdominal organ enlargement or organomegaly nor the suspicion of the presence of any mass and abdominal tenderness. However, the rectal examination revealed a palpable stump with some irregularities at the apex where the surgical staples had been placed during the surgery. He suggested that these irregularities were an artifact from the stapler and that he would like to follow me further after the reversal of ileostomy. He requested further analysis of the blood for CEA test before I return to see him next time.

Plan after recovery from cancer

Several issues are considered in patients' plan after treatments and these include diagnostic records and received treatments; the caring they undergo after the release from the hospital; follow-ups by the family doctor and designated nurses to ensure all heath needs are met; monitoring and preventing the sickness recurrence; and ways to manage the treatment side effects and to deal with psychological and emotional effects of being diagnosed with cancer. Moreover, the plan describes how often one should have a checkup and what tests he will take for the future, and involves the cancer screening process for family members particularly the children. Biologically, my children constitute my close kinship having a high level of genetic relatedness and closer consanguinity to me. Hence, they are also at high risk to inherit similar sicknesses from me. To prevent them from developing the same cancer and from it reaching higher stages of development, it was strongly recommended that my children be monitored and screened for signs of colorectal cancer as earlier as possible—and that should take place at least 10 years before they attain the age at which I was diagnosed with it. To my side, I should continue watching for recurrence of similar symptoms I had initially experienced prior to the disease diagnosis like abrupt weight loss, anal bleeding often with mucus in the stool and internal anal itching, nausea and loss of appetite, and unusual abdominal swelling and acute discomfort. It was also recommended that I should call upon my primary care provider—our family doctor—for an alert on the urgent need to activate and recommend for upcoming tests or treatments as well as to discuss other health issues such as some abnormal long lasting symptoms like numbness.

Family Doctor

I met our family doctor, the primary care provider, as recommended to review my health and discuss the future plan. Before the meeting, I called to the Oncologist's office to find out whether my future plan of action has been released. The nurse who replied to my telephone call indicated that not yet but the plan will have to be first discussed with the Oncologist before sending it to your family doctor. By the time we met, the family doctor was still expecting to get the proposed plan as the Oncologist's nurse had outlined previously. Unfortunately, the plan had not reached her office yet. The first issue I raised, however, was that of persistent numbness symptoms resulting from chemo-radiation treatments particularly on the toes and feet. She indicated that this may take a long time to recede as it has been observed with several other patients. But meanwhile, she prescribed Vitamin B_{12} to be taken daily as a preventive measure to help recover the comfort and relief from the symptoms. She also discussed the need for me to keep up with the implanted bladder stent for an extra 6-month period after which the urologist could change it. The issue for the time of ileostomy reversal to the natural anus was also among the matters the doctor brought out. The intension for raising this was for her, she said, to consult with the surgeon to determine when pre-operative tests and the surgery will be conducted. I left the office after she had conducted some physical examinations of the mouth, the neck surroundings and the abdomen. She said all looked fine.

Ottawa Regional Cancer Foundation

I drove to the Regional Cancer Foundation office with my spouse a week after I met with our family doctor. Our visit was to meet with any of the coaching staffs for advice on which of the various events the center provides that could suit my case and to which I could register. The assistant at the front desk asked that I introduce myself and explain the problem which has brought me to the center. After providing all the details about my sickness and related treatments and tests as well as the test results, she explained the various programs that are offered at the center and asked which ones I would like to follow. She handed over a folder with the various activities and took us for an orientation of the building. Then, I went through all the activities and realized that the most appealing to me at that time were the introduction to massage therapy; coping with cancer and colorectal cancer support group; positive thinking; light and lively exercise; and eating right.

Personally, I found the place as my home away from home and a platform where hospitality and care harmoniously blend to satisfy cancer survivors' needs. It is a place where joy and hope to return to one's normality meet; where one could find abundant opportunities for body and soul enhancement and relaxation. The Regional Cancer Foundation's dedication is to help cancer patients who have survived the different treatments and their family to sustain the survivorship and reduce the suffering and the potential risk of death due to cancer capitalizing on the expertise of available professional staff and several other resources. It also taps on the knowhow from numerous specialists from local hospitals as well as other supportive care groups and researchers in town to implement the cancer awareness and education programs. Workshops and seminars are also conducted by world renowned specialists to provide first-hand information on cancer to patients and their family to enlist them with relevant knowledge from early signs of the disease, on how it could be diagnosed and treated to the monitoring of symptomatic signs that might prompt its recurrence. The survivorship care is offered through one-to-one cancer coaching using health and wellbeing issues to imbed in cancer-survived patients and family practical skills to improve their health and enhance their quality of life.

The coaching process is structured through 45 minutes sessions on average as per the needs that are identified by survivors and their family, often with the following objectives:

1) "Help identify issues to be worked on,
2) Explore motivation and readiness,
3) Make decisions on wellness goals and/or issues,
4) Generate a plan,
5) Identify and address potential barriers, and
6) Review confidence and reinforce access to personal, the center and community resources."

The planned programs that are generated will often include different activities which are selected by survived-patients and family and delivered in group of participants working together with a coach. The program activity could be delivered as a course focussing on a variety of needs tailoring to cancer survivors and caregivers. This type of activity provides support, education and practical skills in various areas of the disease such as its management, nutrition, physical exercise, memory and concentration, stress management, and emotional wellbeing etc. As I was attending activities to which I registered, I regain peace of mind and the body. This came about mainly because of interaction with other survived patients with whom we shared common pain and distress. As such, I will inevitably recommend any cancer patient to adopt the center for post-cancer survivorship advice and management.

Sharing the good news with friends

After receiving the good results of the CT scan of the abdomen and pelvis and that of the chest X-ray following the medication with the 12-cycle chemotherapy treatment and the surgery, I also updated friends on the progress I have made on my health. I wrote:

Dear Friends,

Re: Unforgettable October 12, 2012

Greetings to all from Canada and how are you doing? It is this last Friday that my spouse and I met with my Oncologist doctors to find out what transpired from this month CT Scan of the abdomen and pelvic as well as the chest X-Ray and the blood analysis. Upon arrival in the room, the Oncologist open my file and said all the tests were very good. The screening of scan photos revealed no signs of cancer in the body. He declared me as a new cancer survivor with recommendations to eat well particularly vegetables and fruits, and exercising. I cried with joy and thanked them greatly for their efforts and willingness to save my life. The Hospital Cancer center has now released me regarding the cancer treatment and referred me for a post-treatment follow up to our family Doctor for the next 5 years also with a number of recommendations to do including the body scanning in the first 6 months and thereafter each year. The Oncologist also requested that I contact the Cancer Foundation Center for a training on the "Wellness Beyond Cancer Program" that provides support and guidance once cancer treatment is completed. I am so glad of the outcome and will follow step by step the hospital advice to avoid the disease recurrence. Once again I want you all to know that words are currently lacking to express my gratitude for your support during that time which has been so hard.
Muimba.

Again as before when I had informed them about the colorectal cancer I was diagnosed with, several of the friends from around the globe responded either by telephone calls, electronic mails or by writing postal cards. Some of the few cheerful letters I received clearly demonstrated how happy they were with my recovery from the sickness and all were wishing me a good health. They include:

30/08/2012
Dear Dr Kankolongo

It is great to hear of the news on your recovery progress so far. May Jehovah continue to give power beyond what is normal for a speed recovery. Greetings to the family.
Phil Ng'andwe.

29/08/2012
Dear Dr Muimba

I am glad to hear that you are responding well to the treatment. With God everything is possible. We will continue praying for you. Good day and God bless you.
Stephen Syampungani.

October 14, 2012

How fantastic!! Muimba, we are so happy for you!!!
Neil Rowe Miller.

October 15, 2012
Muimba:

Your message brings great joy also to us. It is evident that your great determination intersected with skilled medical care and that you are a "survivor" despite the long odds. That is truly wonderful news. Take care of yourself. Again, your news is great to hear.

Stella Coackley.

October 15, 2012
Muimba,

Excellent news. What a relief after so much hardship. Florence and the children must be even happier than we are if that is even possible. I almost didn't see this news since my hotmail account was supposedly acked and I could not access it until today. I will email you from gmail next time. Hugs to all,
Diane Allin Florini.

20/12/2012
Dear Muimba

It is sad to hear that a friend of mine has been suffering so much and I have not really been aware of this. At the same time I am happy that you were able to pull through and have made it for now. So good that you have somehow recovered, and I wish you all the best of health and courage for the next steps. This disease is not easy and one needs a lot of courage and help to find some relieve. When I read your plight my request seems to be so minor. Kindest regards, Kerstin.

09/01/2013

Glory and honor be unto our God! Indeed, God does wonders. I thank Him for your healing process. May His name be praised forever. Cheers! Martin.

My sense of the responses from friends was that impression they all truly cared about me and they wanted me back with them again. Their words were inspiring and full of truthfulness and hope. Their writings completely changed my feeling over the circumstances I was going through.

CHAPTER XI
REVERSAL OF ILEOSTOMY

It is really the Lord's grace that my surgeon realised during the surgery for tumor removal that I will benefit more from the reversal of the loop colostomy—a supposed external permanent pouch through which the stool and gas should be released—to an ileostomy, a temporary bag of the same function, and then to the natural anus.

Several months have elapsed since the previous surgery which led to the change of colostomy to a left-sided loop ileostomy and the report that there was no longer a cancerous tumor in my body after the adjuvant chemo-radiation treatment. As a result, the loop ileostomy needed to be reversed to the natural anus through surgery as also more other follow up tests were to be performed to establish the status of the colon.

Surgery for reversal

During a consultation on the state of the wound from the last surgery, the surgeon outlined that some more tests are required prior to the ileostomy reversal. An appointment was set for an endoscopy examination in the radiology department at the Civic Hospital using a Hypaque enema and flexible sigmoidoscopy. The examination of the colon profiling using a minute camera inserted in the colon through the anus went well without any complication. It revealed no evidence of narrowing of the bowel and a breakdown along the site where intestines were merged. Moreover, there were no abnormal overgrowths and any obstruction throughout the colon conduit. CT scans of the abdomen, the pelvis and the thorax without intravenous contrast were also performed. The abdomen and the pelvis were scanned from the diaphragm to the lateral boundary of the pelvic outlet known as ischial tuberosities without contrast because there was no peripheral venous access. Images showed that the stent was still in place extending from the renal pelvis to the urinary bladder. There was no enlargement of the kidney organs that collect urine also known as bilateral hydronephrosis. However, there appeared to be a mild right renal cortical atrophy but the left kidney was preserved. The perirectal and presacral fibrosis were dense, uniform and they were extending cranially along both the sidewalls of the pelvis and more so, on the right side. It is this extension that was causing the ureteric obstruction. Similarly, there was no worrying enlargement of nodular solid masses or lymph nodes. The fluid collection that was previously observed had resolved and the midline of the incision that was partially left open during the surgery had also healed. The lower quadrant loop ileostomy was found to be satisfactory.

The urinary radiograms showed that the bladder had collapsed and that there was a diffuse wall thickening resulting from the numerous complications I suffered from the radiation therapy to the pelvic tumor also known as radiation cystitis. Though the seminal vesicles appeared distorted and somewhat obscured by the adjacent fibrosis, they were however normal and so was the prostate. There were no focal hepatic lesions on the liver and no calcified gallstones that could induce the gallbladder inflammation often resulting from the obstruction of the cystic duct known as cholecystitis or biliary obstructions on the biliary tree. Moreover, the scans showed that the pancreas was normal and that there were now some small para-aortic nodes as compared to large nodes which were previously observed.

It was observed from the thoracic examination that there was no pericardial effusion in the heart and all the systemic and pulmonary vessels were normal. However, there was still that small 3-mm nodule beneath the pleural space on the right lung base as observed during the previous examinations. Otherwise, the remainder of the lung parenchyma was normal apart from the minimal collapsed of the lung that had been resulting in its incomplete expansion. The diaphragm was normal too. There was no presence of any suspicious osseous or soft tissue lesion in the skeleton. But there was a soft tissue nodule with fat measuring about 5 mm in comparison to 7 mm previously observed on the right side around the breast. The radiologist pointed out that the presence of this central fat within the nodule is essential in keeping with benign lymph nodes. Importantly, results revealed that there was no so ever any evidence suggesting the spread of cancer to other organs and tissues in my thoracic body. The result of blood analysis for CEA was excellent. My appetite and body energy were reasonable and I was actively engaged in physical activities such as walking to keep up with my fitness. I did not have any coughing, shortness of breath and change in bowels.

Three months following the notification of the test results, it was time for the surgery. As similar to previous surgeries, I went through the pre-admission checkups at the Ottawa General Hospital where the operation was to be performed. I met with the surgeon for the signing of the consent form. I was informed about the rationale for the surgery to reverse the ileostomy to the natural anus and related risks such as the potential of wound infection; small bowel obstruction; development of a scar tissue on the incision; bleeding and possible injuries to other body organs and structures. After the explanation, I was given a chance to ask any questions. My only concern was about the timeframe for the returning of the normal bowel movements following the surgery. I was informed that in most cases, the majority of patients are pleased with their bowel function although this may never be exactly as what it was prior to the colorectal cancer infection. In addition, the surgeon continued that the healing progress may take up to two years, though for some patients it takes only a few weeks after the surgery. After analysing the benefits resulting from the surgery, I signed the informed consent form and filled out a health questionnaire. I was told I will be contacted for the date of the surgery which could take place no earlier than June 2013. I left the hospital very happy that the pouch I was carrying everywhere will finally be removed.

A month had passed since then. I received a letter from the hospital admitting department notifying me about the ileostomy closure with my surgeon. The location of the surgery was indicated as well as the procedures I had to follow for bowel preparation a week before and the day of the surgery. However, the exact date for the operation was still unknown. Specifically, the noticed underlined the need for me to stop taking drugs such as aspirin and any other types of blood thinning medications one week before the surgery and to contact the admitting department in case I was on injectable blood thinner. I was also instructed to have my normal foods the day before the procedure, but to drink only clear fluids—water, clear fruit juices such as apple and white grape, clear broth soups, any kinds of flavor plain jell-o, clear pops such as ginger-ale and 7-up, tea and coffee without milk, and Gatorade—after dinner. However, clear fluids intake could continue until three hours before the surgery.

Two days after I received the notice for the procedure and for the preparation of the bowel, I had a telephone call from the hospital specifying the exact date of the surgery. It was to take place in April 2013. I reported to the hospital early morning on the indicated day, and was immediately called to follow one of the attending nurses. She took me to an isolation room—since my name in the hospital system is still showing that I carry bacterial infection despite the clearance from the Hospital Infectious Disease Department—where vital signs and other related health issues were recorded. After about 30-45 minutes of waiting, I was taken to the operating room on a stretcher. As per usual procedure, the stretcher was briefly kept in the corridor to allow for the room to be ready. While in the corridor, a nurse provided again instructions on the procedure and collected additional information on my health mainly whether I was allergic to any medication. Then, I was transferred to the room where I was placed supine on the operating table. Again, the surgeon explained that the surgery will commence after you have been intubated under anesthesia. The physician in charge put the IV in one of the veins on my left hand after which he said they were now putting me to sleep. What follows is what the surgeon explained to me few days following the recovery after surgery and hospitalization in the inpatient ward.

She reported that following the anesthesia, a Foley catheter was placed in my bladder. Then, the ileostomy appliance was removed and the area of its attachment (Fig. 19) aseptically washed. Thereafter the anterior abdomen was prepped and draped, the skin incised around the ileostomy using a No. 15 blade knife and antibiotics intravenously administered. After this, the surgeon made another circumferential incision down to the subcutaneous tissue using a sharp No. 15 blade scalpel in order to create an adequate plane between the loop of ileum and the surrounding tissue, the fascia, the rectus muscle and the peritoneum. Once the ileum loop was completely freed circumferentially, it became possible for the team to have a view that I did not have any incisional hernia around the stoma. By the time they reached the peritoneal cavity, they checked for any loops of small bowel that could be adherent to the peritoneum in that location but realized that there were only few adhesions that they easily incised the attachments circumferentially.

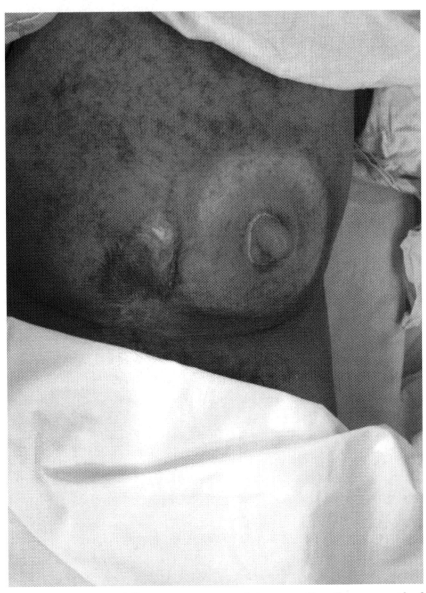

Figure 19. Stomatal ileostomy on my abdomen after the removal of the appliance bag

Since no further adhesions were found, they then divided the scar tissue between the two loops to release the multiple small benign nodules from the afferent basal cells on limb. Similarly, they divided the mesentery between the two loops to create a side-to-side functional and end-to-end anastomosis between the two loops of the small intestine. This was achieved by a single fire of the GIA 80 mm stapler on the portion of the intestine laying opposite to the mesenteric also known as the antimesenteric border of both loops. A second firing was also made to transect the ends and close the open lumens to allow for an adequate anastomosis. Thereafter, a single No. 3-0 Vicryl suture was placed at the apex and the transverse staple line run over again with a similar suture to decrease the chance of a leak. The lumen was placed back in the abdomen after it was found to be adequate following the anastomosis inspection. The inspection they carried out revealed no evidence of any compromised integrity. The incision was then longitudinally closed with interrupted No. 1-0 Maxon in a figure-of-eight fashion and the skin horizontally closed with staples, leaving a small opening in the center (Fig. 20) to be packed with sterile Gauze during wound cleaning and dressing.

The moment the surgery was completed, about two hours later, dressings were applied on the stoma area and the surgeon informed my spouse of the success of the operation that I had tolerated well. Then, I was transferred to the post-anesthetic unit in stable condition for the recovery. When I opened eyes after I fully gained back all my vital signs, I realized I did not bear any external pouch on my abdomen but rather there was now a whitish dressing at site where the ileostomy pouch was prior to the operation. I spent almost 1 hour in the recovery room before I was transferred to my inpatient ward room in the 7th floor of the hospital. As usual, I had routine daily visits by resident doctors and nurses. They all performed professionally as during other times of my previous hospitalization periods. Four days later, I was discharged after I had gradually met several milestones such as ambulatory ability, self-postoperative pain management or analgesia, active bowel function and eating tolerance of some low residue foods. I was very confident of myself and happy to return home not bearing an external pouch serving as an artificial anus. As I was leaving the hospital, strict instructions were given that I call upon the surgeon in about three to four weeks later for a

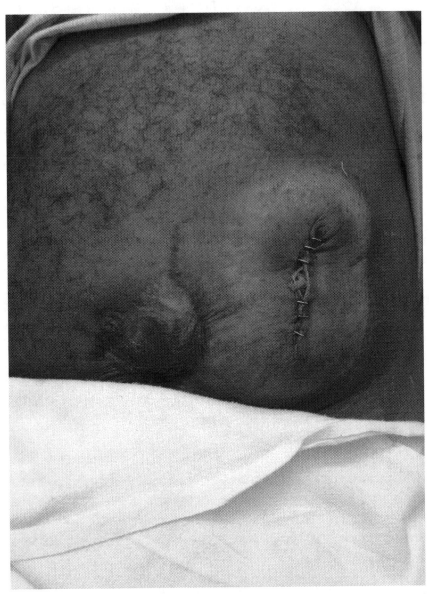

Figure 20. The closed stoma incision with staples leaving a small opening in the center for packaging of the gauze

follow up visit, to initially keep up with liquid foods and gradually change to a solid diet, and to avoid dehydration. The CCAC office was also contacted to follow up with my home care after surgery mainly the wound cleaning and dressing as well as the removal of the staples after well specified days. I fully followed all the steps just as I was instructed.

Gas passing and bowel movement

During the various routine visits by doctors and nurses while I was in the hospital ward, they always asked whether I was now able to eat, pass gas and feel any bowel movement. Since I was still on liquid diet during those first days following the reversal surgery, passing gas and feeling abdominal bowel movement were just minimal. As days passed by, my diet was gradually also changed to solid food which I managed to consume three times a day. This time, the bowel movement phenomenon became common and regular pushing me to regularly go to the toilet and release some stool through the anus although in liquid form. This liquid-like stool continuous until when I was released from the hospital and nearly two months later while at home. Then the solid and consistent stool suddenly commenced to form but it was still accompanied by a liquefied mucus-like substance during its discharge. However, the main problem of my concern was how to control the unexpected continence or my ability to voluntary regulate fecal discharge due to the weakening of the sphincter muscle—on the fringe of the anus—as a result of not working for the last two or so years. However, I recall the surgeon saying during our discussion that this takes some times which may exceed even one year for the muscle to return to normal. To mitigate this, attending nurses initiated an aggressive training exercise for perineal strengthening which I continued on myself at home and anywhere when sitting, walking or driving. The exercise consists of holding as tight as I can my anal canal as if I was refraining from expelling gas or urine for few seconds, relaxing for another few seconds and repeating this several times during the day. Similarly, buttocks squeezing could also provide additional pelvic strengthening that could allow for deferring the bowel movement at a time other than when it is felt. Repeating regularly this exercise somehow assisted in the self-regulatory process of the bowel movement by the sphincter muscle about four months after the surgery.

Wound healing

Visiting doctors and ward care nurses also worried much about several other health issues while I was still in the hospital. Among these were the slow evolution of the healing of the surgery wound and the management of the acute pain I was enduring after the surgery. The question about the pain and the location where this was felt always came about whenever they came to the room. If I had pain, nurses immediately provided necessary medications, either through oral intake or by injection, as prescribed by resident physicians. As part of their duty, nurses also continued cleaning the wound and surrounding areas, and changing the packed gauze and covering it with fresh dressings every day. They also regularly monitored it to prevent potential microbial infection. Nevertheless, I was discharged from the hospital a week after the surgery considering doctors' assessment that everything was functioning well enough to continue with homecare. It took about a month for a complete closure and healing of the wound (Fig. 21). The surgical wound was completely sealed off but the abnormal swelling of the whole area where the ileostomy was in the abdomen constantly disturbed my mind although I knew, from the surgeon's statement that it will stay there for a long time. The other major problem I encountered after the wound had sealed off was still the uncontrollable stool movement. Although this had slightly improved it often occurred without my knowledge particularly during night times when sleeping leading to it spoiling my pyjamas and bed sheets. I had to wear nappies just as babies and change them regularly when they are spoiled. But, the urinal flow was normal due to the implant stent.

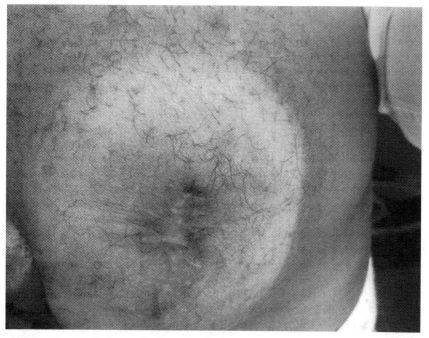

Figure 21. Complete closure of the wound 1 month after surgery leaving behind a swollen area at the site of the ileostomy

Changing the stent

The stent that was inserted between the bladder and the right ureter to facilitate the evacuation of the urine from the kidney to the bladder has been in place for more than 6 months. It was time for it to be replaced with a new one as the Urologist has prescribed. Just a week after I was discharged from the hospital following the surgery, the urology department called to indicate that the time has been set for the stent replacement. I replied that the Urologist should first evaluate my health status and physical fitness for the procedure since the surgery wound from the ileostomy reversal had not completely healed and I was still recovering from the operation. Moreover, I stated that I was just from being discharged from the hospital a week ago. After assessment, the urology department called again a day later to indicate that the procedure has been postponed to another date to be announced at a later time.

A month has elapsed when a new date was fixed. I went through the planning process of the outpatient preparation a week before the procedure. Details of the procedure and how to be prepared for it were given. As usual, these included things to be done the day before the procedure such as eating light food and drinking clear fluids; the morning of the procedure such as taking my usual medications like blood pressure pills; and the morning of the procedure including things I should not bring with me at the hospital and those I should particularly the presence of an adult person to take me back home after the procedure. This person is necessary as I will still be unable to drive on my own within a period of at least 24 hours following anesthesia. Instructions were also given about my care at home mainly on the control of the pain that might ensue after the procedure as well as on the follow-up appointments with the Urologist. Then, I was provided with potential risks that could result from the procedure. After these explanations, I signed the consent form. I was sent to the laboratory for blood and urine analysis, and the heart test. Three days later, I received a telephone call from the urologist office that the culture of my urine showed again infection by Enterococcus bacterial species. As a result, I was prescribed the antibiotic ampicillin to be taken for 10 days, one tablet in the morning and another in the evening. The heart test was normal. From the blood analysis, the CEA was normal while the creatinine was high, and both the white and red blood counts were normal. The fluoroscopy image after injection of the contrast into the ureter in order to visualize the ureter and kidney or the retrograde pyelogram showed a double-J stent well coiled in the right renal pelvis.

On the day of the procedure, my spouse drove me to the hospital. I reported to the front desk of the Surgery Day Care Unit early in the morning before the indicated time.

The first question by the secretary
in charge that day was about the
adult person who will be escorting
me home after the procedure. As my
spouse was not with me at that time
because I left her down looking for a
place to park, I replied "she will be here
in few minutes after she has parked the
vehicle."
She then said "unfortunately sir, your
procedure has been cancelled for today."
My reaction was immediate thinking
that maybe the cancellation is because
I was not with an adult person to drive
me back home after the procedure.
I then asked "why?"
She said "all surgeries today have been
postponed because of unexpected
emergencies in the operating rooms due
to a bus accident with a train somewhere
in town. They are many injured commuters
that the hospital has to intervene rapidly.
Because of this situation, she continued, all
other scheduled operations are postponed."

I thanked her and asked for the telephone I could use to call
and inform my spouse about the situation before she follows me
upstairs. I left the place to the entrance of the hospital where I
found her waiting. We drove home and when we reached there,
I immediately switched on the television to listen to the news to
find out about the accident. We were anxious to have this new
not only to found out about the accident that has resulted in the
cancellation of the procedure of replacing the stent but mainly
because of the concern that two of our children also use the same
public transport system to go to school. This is the only common
public bus transport—OC Transpo—in the capital city Ottawa.

The news was repeatedly broadcasted. The accident occurred between the double decked bus and a train and it caused the death of six people while about 34 others were seriously injured in the hospital. Among the dead was the bus driver also residing in the Orléans suburb where we also live. About ten of the injured passengers were in critical condition. Some of the eyewitnesses were reporting that the safety arm of rail line went down just few seconds before the bus was about to cross. Seeing they were in danger, commuters started yelling for the driver to stop before the crash as they saw other vehicles at the road site had stopped. The driver tried his best to stop the bus but was unsuccessful. They said it was too late because they just realised that the bus hit the train forcing it off the tracks. People were bleeding and screaming all-over in the bus, they concluded.

I returned to the Hospital Surgery Day Care Unit two weeks after the accident and I was taken to the operation room in a gown on a stretcher. An anesthesiologist joined me in the corridor to ask few questions about my past medical history and to establish whether I was allergic to any medications. Inside the room, I was prepared and draped in the dorsal position by attending nurses on the operating table; the nurse put the oxygen masque on my nose and connected my body to numerous machines that will be monitoring my vital signs during the procedure. The anesthesiologist inserted the IV-needle in one of the veins on top of my right hand through which I was to be intubated under anesthesia with 2 g of cefazolin. Before falling asleep, the urologist rapidly briefed me on the procedure. During the procedure, a 22-French rigid cystoscope was introduced into the bladder and an Albarran bridge—with a distal gold-plated reflector having a deflecting mechanism—was used to introduce a Bentson wire and a 5-French Flexi-Tip catheter into the bladder. The distal end of the old double-J uteretic stent was then visualized and was quite encrusted. Through the inserted wire, the team attempted unsuccessfully to make an orifice on the right ureter beside the indwelling stent. They then tried using a Glidewire, which was passed through the 5-French Flexi-Tip catheter to cannulate the orifice as well but were still unsuccessful. Using cold cut rigid biopsy forceps, the team then grasped the stent digital end and withdrew it just outside of the penis. The stent distal coil was cut to try to cannulate it with a Bentson wire but this could not still go through. At this point, the stent was completely withdrawn. Surgeons went back into the bladder with the 22-French rigid cystoscope and Albarran bridge, and after numerous attempts they were finally able to cannulate the right uretetic orifice with a 5-French Flexi-Tip catheter and a Glidewire. The 5-French Flexi-Tip catheter was then advanced into the right kidney under fluoroscopy and the Bentson wire was exchanged for the wire that came with the stent. A black silicone 6-French 24 cm long stent was passed over the stent wire with the proximal end coiling in the renal pelvis. The stent wire was then removed and the distal end of the stent coiled nicely in the bladder. Fluoroscopy images were saved after which the bladder was deinstrumented and a Foley catheter was left in place.

I wake up in the Post-Anesthetic Care Unit (PACU) where a nurse was checking my vital signs—pulse, blood pressure, oxygen level, breathing and the pain level. I was given Tylenol pills for pain control. From PACU, I was sent to the Surgical Day Care Unit (SDCU) where the nurse on duty insisted on instructions that I should urinate first for the Hospital to ensure that the stent has not been dislodged or obstructed before deciding on my discharge. This was so because the ureteral stent is supposed to re-establish a normal urine flow from the kidney to the bladder. The nurse also indicated that the stent may cause you to feel like passing urine more often than usual and that it may also cause a burning feeling when passing urine. This was normal as these effects will reduce with time. However, she insisted that I should not worry in case I notice blood in urine. I should just continue drinking more fluids. I was given two large glasses of water to drink and activate the urinating process. About 45 minutes to 1 hour after, I felt that the bladder was nearly full. I requested the urinary in which I released an amount of urine which they estimated to be normal although I was feeling some pain coming out of the urinary system. Discharge documents were immediately signed following this and my spouse was called to take me home. I continued taking the Tylenol pills for the next three days to manage pain. Before leaving the hospital, the nurse insisted that I should call the urology department in case I realize that it suddenly became difficult to urinate and notice either large blood clots in the urine or severe pain, bloody urine after 3 days or develop severe fever.

CHAPTER XII

RESULTS SIX MONTHS LATER

Six months after I was declared free from cancer, the Oncologist indicated that my blood test was unsatisfactory, raising a concern. He recommended for another blood analysis on the same day to allow for a CT scan to assess my health status. The blood and scan results came out perfect but to ensure that there was no cancer resurgence, another advanced scan test called PTE was performed and results also show no sign of cancer in my body.

*P*rior to obtaining the results, six months later, following previous treatments including the ileostomy surgery, various tests were again performed per requests of medical doctors.

Physical examinations by the surgeon

My appointment was set at 9h00 am one day and I left home 1 hour early to be on time at the hospital. Unfortunately, I got blocked in my way because of a very long traffic jump. I will say that the speed of my vehicle that morning was about 1-2 m each 15-30 minutes. The distance which I always cover within about 10 to 15 minutes when the road is clear took me more than 2 hours. I arrived at the front desk around 10h45. While driving so slowly in the traffic, I cried to the LORD.

> I said "Dear LORD, I pray to you for the surgeon to see me regardless of my late arrival and also considering that she might have several other patients to consult. You know why this traffic has just built on the road before I reach the hospital. I leave everything in your hands, Majesty. In the name of our Savior Jesus Christ, Amen! Thank you Jesus," I concluded.

After that prayer, I drove with a sound mind and amazing peace in mind. The time I reached the hospital, I first looked for an empty space in the parking lot to park the vehicle. As I was approaching the area, I Immediately saw an empty spot between two other vehicles where I managed to park mine. I rushed to the hospital building and the place where I had the appointment. As soon as I was in front of the secretary to present my health and hospital green cards, she said "were you trapped in that long traffic?" "Yes," I replied and quickly added that "I hope the surgeon will still see me." "No problem," she answered. She processed my file and asked me to sit and wait for a call.

Just after about 5 minutes later, a nurse called my name and I was directed to one of the examination rooms. A medical student working with the surgeon came and introduced herself that she will do the physical assessment today and she will ask some questions on my health status before the surgeon comes in. She requested that I dorsally lay on the bed. She checked on the abdomen particularly the place of the surgery wound; pushed along it asking me to cough; and using her stereoscope, she checked and verified the heart rate and the respiration in front of and along the chest as well as on the back. The questions she asked were about the time when the ileostomy was reversed and what was this long scar I had below my umbilici. Moreover, she wanted to know if I was eating well, whether I was able to pass gas and the stool, and if the stool was still in liquid form or has been solidified etc. After recording all the details, she asked that I remain on the bed and left. About 15 minutes after, they entered together with the surgeon who also inspected the wound site. The surgeon indicated that the skin color around the place where the surgery wound had been will disappear with time but the slight swelling and deformity where the ileostomy pouch was fixed is going to be permanent. She noticed that I had not developed a quite large hernia and that the ileostomy has healed very well. Then, she asked whether I was able to control the stool movement or still have encountered uncontrolled movement. Yes, I replied by telling her that often the ileostomy was functioning well with about 3 to 4 bowel movements each day. During day times, I properly manage to control bowel movements, but sometimes it is difficult to predict when it occurs particularly at nights when sleeping, culminating on the stool freely running on the pyjama and spoiling bed sheets. She indicated that such accidents were normal as the reconstitution of the rectum often takes long, sometimes up to 2 years, to adjust and return to normal. Further, I informed the surgeon that I could sometimes observed the reconstitution of my original bowel habits but generally, these are still in liquid form. I did not have any problem controlling the release of urine though I have not attempted sexual functions because of some constant pain resulting from the implanted stent. The abdomen was soft and nontender. Otherwise, the surgeon concluded that everything was looking perfect and planned for another colonoscopy test in 6 months to reassess the colon. Few days later, I received a letter of appointment with the date for the test.

CEA test

The test was requested by the radiation Oncologist and this was to be performed two weeks before I meet with him. The period for the test coincided with the time I was just discharged from the hospital following the surgery for ileostomy reversal. I had lost weight and was still very weak and in pain. However, my spouse took me to a local government laboratory near our community where the blood was to be taken. Unfortunately, attempts by three different nurses to obtain the blood from my veins were repeatedly unsuccessful. They complained that my veins were thinner and hiding into the body that it was very difficult to locate them easily. Needle insertion attempts went on from one arm to the other for about 1 hour trying to found a good vein where the blood could be obtained for analysis. The fourth nurse was called in to help. She brought a warm blanket to cover me for about 10 minutes or so after which she tried unsuccessfully to locate the vein on the left arm. Then as she requested for the right arm, I prayed to the LORD for the vein to show up. She went looking around it and immediately, she successfully inserted the needle in the vein showing on top of my right hand. She said "I got it." I looked at the spot and saw the blood slowly flowing into the first vial. When it was nearly full, she removed the vial as well as the needle. Then, she continued shaking the vial with her left hand to avoid the blood from coagulating and affixed a small bandage on the site where the blood was still coming out. She said now I can go back home since the collected blood was enough for the analysis. The nurse in charge of the clinic confirmed to me that results will be sent to your medical doctor in good time before you see him.

Physical examinations by the Oncologist

On the appointment day, the Oncologist arrived and quickly said on to me that I have considerably lost weight. Yes, I accepted adding that I am just from a surgery two weeks ago for the reversal of my ileostomy. He asked when the surgery took place and when I was discharged from the hospital. Then after usual physical examinations, he said the result of the laboratory analysis for CEA was unsatisfactory and this was of a major concern to them. After the explanation, he wrote and gave to me a blood requisition for another CEA analysis to be done on the same day and this time at the hospital. The reason for this CEA test was to ascertain previous findings and to allow for the radiologists to assess whether they could carry out the CT scan six months after I was declared cancer-free. If the CEA result continues to be either very high or below the standard which is unacceptable, the CT scan will not be conducted. He left the room after this statement and I went directly to the laboratory to provide the blood. The hospital laboratory is within the same location where I was meeting the Oncologist. I presented the request and was asked to sit. One of the nurses joined me and searched a vein in my arms. Fortunately, she was able to locate one rapidly. She extracted the blood sample and I left.

When I reached home, my spouse asked how the visit was. I recounted to her all our conversation with the Oncologist including his concern about the unsatisfactory CEA result and the request to repeat the test. "What does it means?" she asked. "I do not know," I answered. I became so disturbed and distressed to the point of flooding my face with weeping and tears mainly because the CEA also constitutes one of the critical tests that could indicate if someone has cancer. I was pushed to the wall, constantly battling in my mind with the doctor's statement that unsatisfactory results are of concern. "Was this pointing to the recurrence of the sickness?" My mind was asking. But I was of a strong opinion, although not completely convinced, that maybe the unsatisfactory CEA result might be due to the weakness of my body following the surgery. The blood was collected few days after I was discharged from the hospital and my body has not fully recovered. Surprisingly, it was not that long the answer to the question I was asking myself came to the fore of my mind.

"This was the devil attempting to sow confusions and build a mountain of obstacles against your faith in the healing power of the LORD."
No! "I said to myself. Satan is a deceiver and a bluffer. I declared that I am a child of God and fully protected by the holly blood of Jesus Christ. By His stripe I am healed."

From that day onward the Holy Spirit talked to me that it was Satan rooming in my mind, I felt a wonderful peace throughout my body. It was the period when I was in the process of writing a chapter of this book on the results six months after I was declared cancer-free. In prayers I asked the LORD what should I write? The answer was clearly given both in mind and in a dream that you have been healed from that colorectal cancer. I saw in a dream the night that followed my visit with the Oncologist a young lady in athletic uniform with ileostomy and surgery wounds, exactly similar to what I had. She was narrating to me that these items she carries and the cancer she suffered from have completely healed. I was so happy for her in the dream mainly that she is healed from cancer. These events prompted my writing in the book the results of CT scan and CEA tests were excellent before even meeting with the Oncologist. I was so confident of myself that I no longer had the sickness. It is gone and I am free from it.

Blood and CT scan tests

Few days later, I received a letter from the hospital that I was booked for a CT scan test for the abdomen and pelvis. I thanked the LORD because this showed that the CEA analysis has turned out to be satisfactory and this is why I have now been asked to go for this test. As I reported to the desk of the secretary in the radiology department situated in Module X, she provided me with those two large glasses of contrast dyes having a bad taste and to be drunk slowly for about 1h30. Before the second glass was empty, the laboratory technician asked me to follow him in the testing room. I was instructed to lay down the face turned up on the scan bed after which the scanning was performed. I left the hospital just after less than an hour.

Test results

My spouse took me to the hospital and she went for her appointment with a lawyer in town. I reported to the secretary desk and she asked that I wait for the nurse call. I was in the waiting space for about 15 minutes when my spouse came back that on her way she stopped to found out the direction but realized the time for her appointment has passed. She called the place and she was told it was too late but she needed to arrange for another appointment time. The nurse called me about another 10 minutes later. My spouse and I followed her up to one of the examination rooms. She checked first my weight before we enter and said it will not be long for the oncologist to arrive. He entered the examination room shortly thereafter, pulled out the copy of the CT scan reports from my file and said: "As compared to the results of the previous test 6 months ago, scan images of the abdomen and pelvis with intravenous and oral contrast did not reveal anything matter of concern such as focal masses or ductal dilatation and increased convexity that would suggest any metastatic disease. Additionally, he continued that the bladder thickening was unchanged but there were some nodular thickening at the root of the small bowel mesentery measuring about 11 x 8 x 20 mm and some prominent small lymph nodes in the vicinity of the peritoneum area with increased size probably either as a result of the recent surgery or early spread of the disease in my body. Moreover, there were no upper abdominal or pelvic lymph nodes, but obvious cortical thinning of the right kidney and some enhancement of the layer of tissues lining the urinary tract were observed but these were consistent with the secondary chronic obstruction. The left kidney was normal whereas the right one was atrophic with mild enlargement of some parts of the kidney. The scan of the thorax with intravenous contrast showed that the heart, systemic vessels, the esophagus, diaphragm, pulmonary vessels, trachea and bronchi were all normal. The size and distribution of lymph nodes in the area directly under the joints around my shoulder known as axillae, the central compartment of the thoracic cavity or mediastinum and both hila—areas through which ducts, nerves, or blood vessels enter and leave body glands or organs—were all also normal. There was no any aggressive osseous lesion on the skeleton and soft tissue. However, a presence of unchanged tiny soft tissue nodules was noticed in the pre-pectoral fat bilaterally which would suggest a likely of benign intrapulmonary lymph node.

As before, the physical examinations showed no palpable cervical and supraclavicular adenopathy and that my chest was found to be clear without any noise in the stethoscope. The heart sounds were normal and there were no palpable abdominal organomegaly, masses and tenderness although the abdomen was somewhat distended. The blood analysis showed that nearly all the blood parameters tested—white and red blood counts, hemoglobin and hematocrit, platelet count, absolute neutros, magnesium, sodium, potassium and calcium—were on the lower side. Nevertheless, the creatinine and CEA levels were very high. He said that the radiologist wasn't sure whether or not the observed small nodularity represented an early metastasis but that he was still very much concerned about the CEA result. To ensure the status of the observed lymph nodes and because of the rising levels of creatinine and the CEA, the radiation Oncologist recommended that I provide again blood for another blood test and also to have another CT scan as well as the advanced scan test called Position Emission Tomography (PET). He suggested having both the standard CT and PET scans combined. PET/CT scan combinations are effective in localizing some suspected areas of abnormal 18F-FDG uptake that will precisely help in the diagnosis and estimates of extent of the disease recurrence. Furthermore, he said that often they are not allowed to request this test for patients on regular basis because of its high cost. In this case, he continued, I wanted to ensure there was no recurrence of cancer in my body. By the way, he asked "did the surgeon perform a complete colonoscopy?" I replied this examination has been planned to take place in the following few weeks from to date but I did not have the exact date of the test. The repeat of the blood analysis resulted in a creatinine value about half below that was earlier obtained while that of the CEA was excellent within the acceptable range.

Positron emission tomography (PET) scan

The PET test uses some radiation to make detailed pictures of the body parts, therefore showing how well the chemistry of the various organs and other tissues function or could be affected by cancer (Colorectal Cancer Association of Canada at http://www.colorectal-cancer.ca/en/screening/pet-cancer/). I praised the LORD for the CT scans of the abdomen and the pelvis again revealed no suspicious signs of a cancerous tumor or presence of any contaminated tissues in the colon. The Majesty is good all the time and glory be to Him, I proclaimed. I thanked the doctor and we went together with my spouse to the laboratory for the blood suction as requested.

A week later after meeting with the Oncologist, I received a call from the Nuclear Medicine department of the Ottawa hospital that the appointment for the PET test has been set for the 27th June 2013 at 8h30 in the morning. Moreover, instructions for the preparation before the test were given specifying that I should not do hard physical exercise two days before the test; I can take my normal medications but making sure they do not contain sugar and I should fasten 6 hours before the appointment time. Meanwhile, I could continue drinking plain water. Regrettably however, I was called a day before the test that I should not report to the hospital as scheduled due to malfunctioning of the machine and that I will be informed of the new date once the PET machine is repaired. The new date was fixed for the 10th of July at the same time as for the first appointment. When I arrived at the hospital on the indicated date, I presented both my health and the hospital green cards to the secretary. After a short search in her computer, she identified my name and went on asking me routine questions to ensure I was the right patient.

"What is your last name?
How do you spell your first name?
What is your birth date?
At which address you reside?
What is your telephone number?" She asked.

I provided an answer to each of these questions. After she was satisfied with my responses, she took me to a lobby where I had to wait for the laboratory technician administering the test. Before leaving, she added that unfortunately they are about 1 hour behind schedule. I should just sit and wait until the time I am called. I sat for about 45 minutes when I became anxious. I went back to the secretary to find out what was going on. She indicated that I should just wait because they have been late because of so many patients before me. Seeing that they were other patient in front of me, I just sat and waited.

About 1 hour later, one of the technicians came and called me for additional questions and explications of the procedure. The questions were about my identity and the exact home address; my medical history including types of past surgeries and cancer treatments I went through; the medications I was currently taking such antibiotics for any infection; if I was allergic to any medication, whether I was diabetic or not; and if I had had any biopsy on any of my body parts during the past two weeks. She informed me that before proceeding with the PET test, she will assess my sugar level which should be at least lower than the target rate of 9 mmol/L often recorded from diabetic patients. To my knowledge, at least 3.6-5.0 mmol/L is considered a normal fasting glucose level. The sugar level test was immediately done with an OneTouch A1C reading meter using the blood sample obtained from the tip of one of my finger. Following a satisfactory result, she then indicated that I will be intravenously infused in my bloodstream—through a IV inserted in one of the veins on top of my right hand—with a radioactive tracer named fluorodeoxyglucose (F-18 FDG). The composition of the tracer includes sugar and a radioactive element that can be rapidly used as a source of energy by cancer cells. As a result, these diseased cells can be easily detected through a PET scan. The scanning consists of an array of detectors that surround the patient when h/she is lying on the machine bed. Using the gamma ray signals that is given off by the injected DG, the test could measure the level of metabolic activity at a site of infection in the body and a computer reassembles the signals into images. In this way, cancer cells will show up as denser areas on a PET scan that are nicely lit up. PET is useful in diagnosing certain cancers because it highlights areas with increased, diminished or no metabolic activity, and offers an effective mean to determine for cancer recurrence. She continued by saying that I will be also given two glasses of a contrast dye for the CT scan which will be combined with the PET analysis. When these tests are combined, they provide a clear picture of internal diseased structures. The scanning will be done from my head to the toes, she concluded.

Then, she asked.
"Do you have any particular question of concern before we proceed with the procedure?"
"Oh yes" I answered.
"What is it?" She asked.
"What might be the potential effects of the radioactive element of the FDG on the patient's body?" I replied.
"As far as I know, this chemical does not have any side effect on the body." She confirmed to me.

"That was the only question I had." I said.
"After you finish drinking the two glasses of the dye, use the toilet on the corner to empty your bladder." She added before leaving the room. She indicated to me the exact direction where patients' toilet was.

She returned few minutes later to the room where I was with necessary needles to be introduced in a vein from any of my arm. She rapidly identified a suitable vein from my left arm into which the IV was successfully inserted. To ensure this was working perfectly, she tried flushing it and sucking the blood from it as usual. Then, the two glasses of the dye was given to be taken each for 30 minutes. Before I started drinking the dye, she pulled the infusion pole to connect the tubing from the saline water bag to the IV to allow for a smooth flow into my body for few minutes first followed by an intravenous administration of about 396.8 MBq of the FDG through the same IV. The saline water, which has the same concentration as the blood, facilitates an easy flow of the FDG into one's blood stream. After both the bags of water and the tracer were empty, which was about 1 hour, I was requested to relax for another 1 hour to allow for the tracer to spread throughout the body blood stream. During this relaxation period, I continued with the sipping of the dye. At the end, I was asked to use the toilet to flush out the bladder for it was full of water before I was taken in the scanning room. Once I was inside, one of the technicians helped to position me correctly on my back on the scan bed and requested that I lie still throughout the procedure (Fig. 22). Before starting the test, I had to open the belt from my pant and pull it down up to the level below the knees. I was covered with warm bed sheets after which the technician left the scanning room to join the other laboratory technician in the adjacent room with the computing and intercom systems. Here, they could easily monitor the patient through a glass window. Within 3 to 5 minutes, the bed was computer-activated. It then slowly moved in and out the machine for nearly 1 hour during

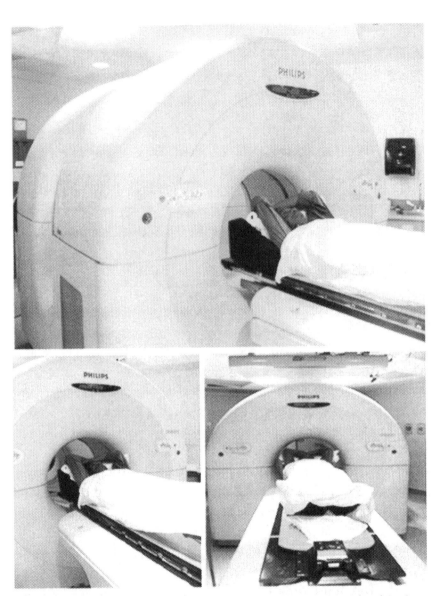

Figure 22. Lying on my back on the PET scan machine bed (top) before being pushed in for the scanning (bottom left and right) at the Ottawa General Hospital in 2013

which it was making buzzing and clicking noises. During this time, a CT scan without intravenous and oral contrast and at low mA levels was acquired for attenuation correction and localization purposes. Subsequently, PET images from the skull base to mid thighs of my body were acquired through the Philips Gemini Dual Exp PET/CT scanner. At the completion of the test, the technician returned into the room to push completely the bed out of the machine. He asked me to wait until the radiologist confirms if the obtained pictures were of good quality for a satisfactory interpretation of the needed information. Few minutes later, I was informed that I should be injected again through the IV with another medication called Lasix which facilitates a proper evacuation of the urine from the bladder to have good pictures. The medication was very effective for I went to the toilet to pass out water four successive times within 30-45 minutes from the time it was injected. I was again taken to the room for the PET test, but this time only for about 10 to 15 minutes. Following this, the CT scan, PET scan and fused images were reconstructed in the right angle along the axis of the body (transaxial), and in both the orthogonal to the transverse or coronal as well as the orthogonal to the transverse and coronal projections, respectively. All the images were finally interpreted accordingly from the HERMES Workstation combining data of the images taken from various sources.

PET/CT scans results

The appointment to meet with both the radiation and chemotherapy Oncologists was scheduled only two days following the test day. I woke up happily that morning for reasons I could not explain myself. After taking a thorough bath, I wore one of my white shirts which is my most preferable outfit, a black trouser and then put on my black shoes which I finely polished the previous night. With this outfit on, I was feeling so self-confident and comfortably evident that I was going to receive good results. This looked so much that day I was awaiting so long. I was very sure the LORD has already healed me and that the result will certainly be very good. I said a short prayer internally thanking the Majesty our God for the healing before I left home. I drove to the hospital singing loud one of the songs playing on the CD. When I reported to the front desk of the module where I was to meet the doctors, I was comfortably smiling. I submitted to the secretary my hospital green card and the health card. She pulled out my file and asked whether I was still living at the same address, which I confirmed. Then, she requested that I should go first to the computer at the waiting space to fill in the ISAAC chart which assesses patients' wellbeing and then wait for a call. I completed the required form and sat down. After about 45 minutes, I was called to follow the nurse to the examination room. When we reached the place, she recorded my weight and asked that I remove clothes and wear the gown. The scale indicated that I have gained 1 kg from the weight I had recorded during the last visit a month ago. She said the doctor will be here very soon and left.

The radiation Oncologist arrived in the room about 30 minutes from the time I was waiting. As soon as he entered, he requested that I lie on the bed for some physical examinations. He was wearing a white gown, traditionally used by medical doctors and was surprisingly also singing happily by whistling maybe one of his favorite songs. He checked my respiration from the front to the back of the chest using his telescope, touched around my neck if there were some lymph nodes, pushed hardly down my abdomen and carefully observed the surgical wound scars. Then, he requested that I lie down on the side to introduce his finger in the anus to check whether or not there were some obstructions in the rectal channel. "All seem to be perfect," he said.

Then he opened my file that he was carrying and went through some papers looking for the page with the PET results. When he saw the page, then he happily said:

> "There is good news for you. The CEA test result was very good. This time it came out normal (about 3.0) compared to 36.0 previously recorded. I think, he pointed out, those later results were not reliable at all. They considerably prompted various questions of major health concerns. But we are now fine with these results. At the end,

he requested that in future I should not use that laboratory for any analysis."

I told him that "I went to this laboratory because I was just from being discharged from the hospital after the surgery for the ileostomy reversal. I was very weak and the wound was still fresh that I could not reach the laboratory at the hospital." He insisted that "all future laboratory analyses should be done only here at the hospital."

He then asked "how was I feeling?"

I said "I was feeling good but that I was anxious to know the result of the PET test I just done two days ago."

Again, he flipped out several pages in the file to have the test report and said when he reached there that he was going to read only the concluding statement which is important:

"The nuclear medicine physician wrote that the analyses of images they obtained show no evidence at all for recurrence of cancer."

I instantly shouted:

"Thank you Jesus; thank you LORD and glory be to you Jesus."

He said "Congratulation for such a good and encouraging result. We are now discharging you for follow up scan tests by your family doctor who should also recommend for the blood and physical tests to be conducted twice a year to be on the safe side. He concluded that he did not see any further role for the radiation Oncologist at this point, but he will be more than happy to see me again should that need arise in future." After this statement he requested that I remained in the room for the chemotherapy Oncologist and left.

Specifically, results of the PET scan showed that there was no abnormal FDG activity in my body as well as the hypermetabolic swelling cervical lymph nodes in the head and the neck that were scanned. Similarly in the chest, there was no focally increased FDG activity within regions where blood vessels and nerves enter, and in the axillae and the lung parenchyma. Lungs were clear and there was no mediastinal lymphadenopathy in the pelvic region. Within the abdomen and pelvis, there was no hypermetabolic mesenteric or retroperitoneal lymphadenopathy. The liver, spleen and adrenal glands all were within normal limits. However, there was significant radiotracer retention within the urinary bladder (Figs. 23) as prior to Lasix administration although there was no significant increase of the FDG activity in the presacral soft tissue density at the anastomosis and in the bones. The radiologist concluded that there was no so whatever evidence of residual or recurrent colon cancer in view of the whole patient body from the skull base to the mid-thigh area.

The chemotherapy Oncologist entered the room about 15-20 minutes later and was comfortably well dressed in a purple suit. He said: "I was briefed that you have very good result from the PET test. Sit on the bed for some physical exam." Which I did. He also checked around the head and the neck, the abdomen and on the feet, and assessed my respiration from the chest, cardiovascular, lymphatic and peripheral systems. Overall, the result was normal. After this he also said:

> "The cancer clinic is going to discharge and refer you again to the Ottawa Regional Cancer Foundation for a period of wellbeing counselling after cancer treatment."

I rapidly replied that "I am already with the Regional Cancer Foundation at Mapple House following your last recommendations which was 6 months earlier when I was declared cancer-free."

"In that case it is alright" he said. Then, I asked about the persistent numbness on the feet that the radiation Oncologist had said it was due to chemotherapy treatment. He said "these types of symptoms will last for sometimes which may be very long

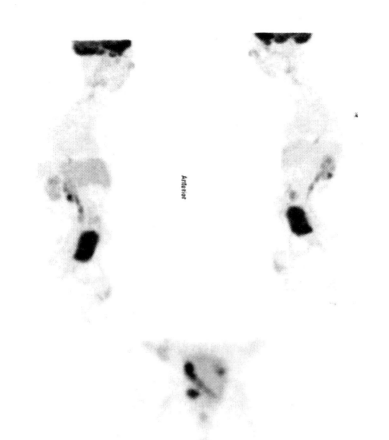

Figure 23. PET scan images of my left and right sides (top) and the pelvis (bottom) projection display showing no areas with abnormal ^{18}F-FDG uptake at the sites of the abdomen and pelvis where the tumor was removed to suggest recurrence of the cancer

and medication to mitigate this?" I asked this because I am currently taking vitamin B12 that the Ottawa Cancer Foundation had recommended it could alleviate the side effect. He replied that "I was not sure whether this will work but after sometimes the symptoms could recede." At this point, he left.

I put back on my clothes and left too. It is at this moment that I felt completely delighted and over-confident that I should now go back to where I left off from my work before I was diagnosed with the sickness. Indeed, I was so happy; feeling very released from the illness stress and relieved from the perpetual anxiety that was bothersome. I said to myself this problem was over for ever although some of its side effects particularly the numbness was still persistent. Overall, I was feeling so well and considered I can perfectly manage this side effect. The question then becomes whether I should now return to my work in Africa as soon as I can. Though my work turned out to be the first priority, I was still concerned about the cost of travelling forth to Africa and back regularly to Canada to report to the hospital for the various forthcoming appointments including CT scan and CEA tests to be done each 6 month as it has been recommended. Just as I was battling in my mind with this idea, I received a devastating letter from my employer terminating my job.

Colonoscopy examination and results

The first post-operative surveillance colonoscopy of the bowel (Fig. 24) was to be performed by the surgeon. I reported to the endoscopy unit on the date of the appointment where the nurse instructed me to remove all my clothes plus socks and shoes. Then, she handed over to me the gown to use during the test and requested that I stay on the bed for the test. She recorded first the blood pressure and several other issues regarding my health history. Thereafter, I was inserted an IV in my right arm through which an anesthesia of 100 g Fentanyl, 10 mg Diazemuls was intravenously injected. The surgeon discussed with me the rationale for the procedure as well as related risks of bleeding and perforation that might result from the test. After the explanation, I signed the informed consent form.

As I initially indicated, I was first placed supine and then positioned lying laterally down on the left side or in the lateral decubitus position after the examination of the abdomen. The physical observation demonstrated a soft non-tender abdomen

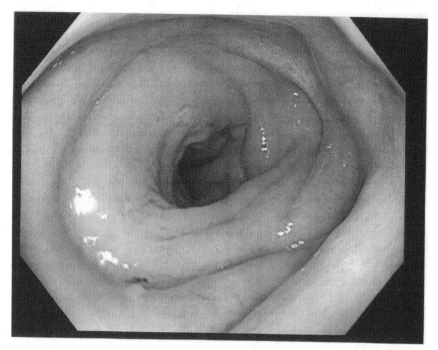

Figure 24. Portion of my colon from the anus indicating that the junction of intestines that were made during surgery to reverse to the normal anus was normal and well healed

also showed that there was not any issue of concern. Then, a miniature camera scope was inserted into the anus and passed up to the beginning of the large intestine with minimal difficulty. The cecum was identified by the presence of an ileocecal valve and the appendiceal orifice. By slowly withdrawing the scope, the surgeon was able to carefully and thoroughly examine the entire colon. At the end of the procedure, which I tolerated well, the scope was slowly removed. It was found that there was no evidence of polyps or mass lesions. The anastomosis was normal and well healed. Following these findings, the surgeon recommended for another colonoscopy to be done in 5 years' time as per current Cancer Care Ontario Guidelines. She also suggested that it was necessary to meet with her again only after 5 years for a follow up colonoscopy. This visit will take place only after the physical examination by our family doctor closer to that time. About one week after the colonoscopy test, I experienced a serious constipation that prompted me to take once again the laxative medication—Dulcolax pill—to stimulate the bowel movement. Though I had a brief relief following the medication intake, the problem recurred but only for a short period. Surprisingly following the constipation, the nature of the stool suddenly changed from liquid to soft consistency. Since that time however, my initial stool habit has taken its normal course. I have undergone the follow up scanning for 2½ years now and results show no sign of cancer.

CHAPTER XIII

LOSS OF MY JOB

> *As I was happy because of the test results showing no cancer in my body, I received a letter from my employer abrogating my contract. The letter came as an unspeakable tragedy adding another heavy load to my already physical and mental suffering from the sickness, surgeries and the side effects of the radio-chemotherapy treatments.*

*J*ust when I was rejoicing the health recovery from the LORD following the announcement of very good test results six months after treatments and surgeries—which were also consistent with those obtained following the 12-cycle chemotherapy regimen—I received a shocking letter from the institution where I was working in Zambia that invigorated my emotional distress.

Abrogation of my contract

The letter indicated, unexpectedly, the termination of my contract due to a very long time being away from work according to the established conditions of service. My contract with the institution was for a three-year period which came to an end at that time the letter was written. I was not given an opportunity to say whether or not I intended to renew it. The letter came as an unspeakable tragedy adding another heavy load to the already physical and mental suffering from the sickness, surgeries and the side effects of the radio-chemotherapy treatments I was enduring. I left my working place in Zambia to Canada with sick leave permission of 6 months for medical attention. As treatment for cancer takes a long time, the sick leave was extended twice. But this time, the institution just decided to end my contract. It was so cruel to bear. The letter read:

3ʳᵈ June 2013
Dear Dr. Kankolongo,

I write to advise that your contract of employment that came into effect on 7ᵗʰ May 2010 expired on 6ᵗʰ May 2013. In view of the foregoing, the Bursar is hereby authorised to pay your accrued benefits less any obligation due to the institution. Allow me on behalf of the Copperbelt University Council to sincerely thank you for the period you served the institution. Yours faithfully,
ACTING REGISTRAR,
Copy to the Vice Chancellor, the Deputy Vice Chancellor, Bursar, Chief Internal Auditor and the Dean, School of Natural Resources.

I loved so much my work more especially the research component continually investigating the nature, and socio-economic and cultural characteristics of smallholder farming systems in Southern Africa. Any way! I considered the matter has come and there was nothing else I could do to change the situation. I showed the letter to my spouse and asked for her advice to respond to it as the matter was so stressful to handle on my own. Because of this, I suddenly felt a complete disruption and bizarre change in my life, and uncertainty in my future. Several questions came into mind such as what was going to happen to my family, often causing overwhelming fear and trembling. Personally, I did not join the University solely for money, but to share with students and co-workers my experience over more than 30 years working on-farm with resource poor small-scale farmers and collaborating with national scientists and NGOs in Southern Africa for agricultural development and poverty alleviation. At the same time, my work also played a central role in my life defining my family process and outcome as well as fulfilling its specific needs and desire. It was the sole source of my financial security, providing for the income needed for my household needs and obligations.

After reading the letter, she outlined to me some key elements I could include in my acceptance response. She advised that these positive elements will serve the purpose of avoiding negative attitude and quarrelsome statements that could show that the termination of my contract was unfair and unlawful treatment since I was away for medical attention. Rather, they will reflect a positive attitude towards the numerous opportunities the institution had offered me to enhance further my skills and capacity, and how working there had also helped in learning new coping strategies. More importantly was her idea of greatly thanking the institution and its entire management for the opportunity that was given to work as one of its staff. She also insisted that I should include in my letter a statement that this was neither the university's fault nor my personal intention to have delayed for so long my return to resume work. I wrote a long letter giving details of the progress on the sickness and on what remains to be achieved. In so writing, I felt fully released from the distress and the continuous thinking about the situation. Thereafter, I called the Ottawa Regional Cancer Foundation for further advice.

Counselling for emotional distress

I explained the reasons for my call over the telephone requesting an appointment to meet with one of the coaching counsellors at the Ottawa Regional Cancer Foundation. Through the discussions, she first raised the point to assess my current health status after medical treatments I received and the survivorship care I went through at the Foundation. Then, I also pointed out about the issue of a considerable emotional distress I was going through following the termination of my employment. I told her that I had been informed that the center was also dealing with such situation. If that was the case, I then believe I could also benefit through your counselling to ease and cope with the emotional distress and the already existing anxiety from the sickness I am going through to enjoy again my life. Following the advice, I obtained an appointment to discuss the issue with the center counsellor. When I walked in, the counsellor took me to her office and said....

"It has been some times since we discussed both on one to one assessment and through emails."
"Yes indeed, I replied."
How have you been with your sickness?"
"Everything looks bright, I replied. I recently did CT scan and PET tests and results of both tests were encouraging. They did not show any sign of cancer in my body." I added.
"That's good news," she pointed out.
"What about treatment side effects—such as numbness—we discussed about last time when we met?" She continued.
I said "I still feeling these remnant effects and I continue taking vitamin B12 as indicated in the document you had given me and also following the prescription by our family doctor."
Then she asked.
"How do you cope with this?"
"I regularly do physical activities such as walking around and also I shared with friends the various issues I continue facing," I replied.

"That's good, because by doing so, you release yourself from the anxiety and stress," she rapidly emphasized.

"What brought you to my office today?" She continued.

I said "I came to seek for advice and emotional counselling."

"What is the problem?" She asked.

I replied "That matter of termination of my employment contract I had indicated during our telephone conversation."

"I see, could you narrate it to me again?" she asked.

I retraced back the situation when I left Zambia for medical attention after I took sick leave for six months which was later changed to one year. After the progress report on my health and the possible date I could return to resume my job was sent to Zambia by my Oncologists, the institution first reduced my salary to half saying this will be reinstituted upon my return to work and then terminated my employment at the end of my contract. When I finished, she raised the question of whether we had some financial difficulties in our household. No, I replied. We were still coping well with the situation although only relying on my spouse's income to keep up with our daily household's needs. She informed me that in case of any difficulties with our finance, there were a number of organizations in Ottawa which provide financial assistance and that she was willing to contact them on my behalf. However, she continued, it is always preferable that we consider reviewing our family budget as a way of cutting down some unnecessary expenditure. I replied that we have not sat to go through items of high priority; my spouse always carefully looks up on this to ensure only the important items were first covered. Then, she asked "whether I have been paid terminal benefits by my employer." "No," I replied. The institution had requested that before the payment of terminal benefits is effected, I should first nominate a co-worker as my representative to undertake on my behalf the clearance for any of the university properties I obtained and left in the office at the time I left Zambia on 23 April 2011 for medical attention to Canada up to 3 June 2013 when my contract ended. The institution also agreed that the payment will be made once the clearance process is completed, which I will be informed through my representative. In fact, the clearance was completed by mid-August 2013 but up to this time—end of August—I have not heard anything about the payment. She loudly pointed out that I will have to vigorously and closely follow this matter and repeatedly call or write to them because some organizations will always tend to delay payment if the beneficiary is far away and do not pressurise them. I agreed for the advice to follow up on the payment.

Recreating my future

From this issue, the coach moved on to trying to know if I was doing my best to secure for another employment. "Yes," I responded. I have realized at this moment that there was no way I will return to Zambia after treatments to resume my job. This job was over. I will have to fight back and find another way of life here in Canada. Up to this time, however, I never taught another job was needed since the main focus was only about my health. Nevertheless, being now laid off from the job of lecturing to students that I loved so much and for which I had deployed most of my energy really triggered my thinking for the future. Various good and bad moments during decades of my work started navigating in my mind. I saw myself when I was in different farms discussing with smallholder farmers and collecting samples; in laboratories diagnosing plant diseases and viewing microorganisms through microscopic observations; in classrooms lecturing to students or in office developing new academic curricula; in faculty committee meetings deliberating on students' grades or discussing about any departmental issues of concern; at international workshops presenting papers; at training course as a resource person to build on the capacity in research for national collaborators; performing consultancy works for international organizations; writing proposals to look for funds for own or future collaborative research and writing scientific articles for publication etc. For me, completing these tasks was just one of the most rewarding feelings and achievements I have accomplished. From the perspective of my career, I was surely convinced that I was well prepared and equipped to contribute in the agricultural sector in Canada or anywhere in the world having a graduate degree in agricultural science and with my long history of field experience working in research with national scientists and outreaching to farmers in sub-Saharan Africa. My vision has always been to serve farmers and this vision strongly encouraged me to get back on my feet and reach out again on my personal and professional pursuits to accomplish something far beyond what has been in my past.

I indicated to the coach I was consulting about the emotional stress following the end of my last contract to seek for the way forward. However as a result of this development, I have been searching and applying for employment to several institutions of interest both here in Canada and abroad; but I was just waiting for any invitation for interview. She suggested that while waiting for a call, I should also know that there are several organizations in Canada that offer counselling and training to job seekers as well as seminars for interview preparation and review of résumés to fit the Canadian context. Because I was so much interested on knowing more about these centres, particularly those close to my community in Orléans, she provided me with few addresses I could contact on my own free time. At the same time, I was also interested in temporally filling in for some volunteer work at either any of the Canadian companies dealing with agricultural activities or the Ottawa General Hospital assisting other cancer patients. This activity would lift up my moral and help for my interaction with the local community after a long time in and out of the hospital. The main question was how could I work and perform in a setting in which I have not been exposed to before. To confront the various issues challenging people in a new environment, I necessarily needed to be part of the Canadian community. Therefore, a volunteer activity for at least a short period particularly in agriculture would be beneficial to my experience. It was important to find an organization that could accept me at least for a short period for volunteer work. She agreed with my suggestion and indicated that the Ottawa Regional Cancer Foundation was looking for volunteers to perform different tasks. She went to the secretary desk to download related forms that she handed over to me to apply in case I was interested. I left the office and immediately returned home. Shortly after, I went through the volunteer opportunity and application forms but realised that the duties and responsibilities for the custodian volunteer the Cancer Foundation was looking for did not limit just to the maintenance of the surrounding such as gardening but it also involved the cleaning of the kitchen, rooms and all the public areas, and arranging the space for meetings and other program activities. I felt these tasks were too demanding and beyond my capacity at this time when I was just recovering from a devastating sickness.

Contact with Cornell University

As I was still meditating about the custodian volunteer at the Regional Cancer Foundation, I suddenly remembered suggestions during a conversation that I should feel free to indicate to my former supervisor at Cornell University in case I need to be introduced to his colleagues in Plant Pathology in Canada. I said to myself this was a good idea. I quickly then dropped on to him a short email outlining my interest that he should contact these scientists on my behalf. I received his reply the following few minutes asking for my CV, which I quickly forwarded to him. Thereafter, he circulated it to some of his colleagues particularly those in the Agriculture and Agro-Food Canada (AAFC) and at some local universities. His letter read as follow:

Date: October 27, 2013 10:08:33 PM EDT
To: …..
Subject: Introducing Dr. Muimba Kankolongo

Dear Colleagues at ECORC:

"I hope that all is well with each of you. I want to make you aware of a job seeker who lives in the Ottawa area and who is an outstanding plant pathologist, agricultural researcher and teacher.

I have attached the C.V. of Dr. Muimba-Kankalongo. Muimba completed his Ph.D. with me in 1991 working on resistance in maize to anthracnose. He has had a distinguished career as an agricultural scientist in Africa including as a member of the faculty of Copperbelt University in Kitwe, Zambia since 2004. Muimba become seriously ill a few years ago and moved to Ottawa for the superior medical care available in your city. After years of complex surgery and convalescence, Muimba has now received a clean bill of health from his doctors, he has regained his energy, and he hopes to find employment in the Ottawa area in some position where he can contribute his considerable skills to agricultural advancement. I should add that during Muimba's long convalescence in Ottawa he wrote an absolutely astounding and fully illustrated, 470-page book that will serve as guide to crop production practices for smallholder farmers in southern Africa. Muimba's strongest interest and strengths are in crop field research assessing disease resistance and other management methods. He also has a strong background in food spoilage and mycotoxins. Muimba is a permanent resident of Canada and resides in Orleans, ONT with his wife and children. He can be reached by phone (613-837-3504) or email (mambayeba@ yahoo.com). I would consider it a personal favor if you could make Muimba or me aware of any employment opportunities relevant to his skills in the Ottawa region -- and those opportunities could be in government, industry, or academia. Should you have an opening for a researcher in one of your programs, you would find Muimba to be a hard-working and talented scientist. Please feel free to forward this message to your colleagues. I appreciate any leads or advice that you can offer Muimba.
Very best regards,"

Shortly after the letter was circulated, I received a number of encouraging copies of the feedbacks they wrote to him among which, one was from the Eastern Cereal and Oilseed Research Centre in Ottawa of the AAFC offering a volunteer work for some times. This attracted my attention very much. I responded favorably to it and was called for further discussions. I met with the program Manager about two days later and we agreed that I feel in various forms including those for the security check and the Research Participant Agreement between the institution and the applicant. By signing the forms, I will whereby be allowed an opportunity to work in a Canadian research program and gain knowledge in corn breeding and pathology. During my attachment, I will be working with the program leader and his staff to learn about the major diseases of corn in Canada and how the crop is selected and breed for resistance to these diseases. Moreover, I will be assisting with the evaluation of disease resistance and then spend some time in the laboratory learning some culture techniques for the various corn pathogens in Canada. After a security check, which took about two weeks, I was called to sign volunteer work forms at the human resources office, and to obtain the motor vehicle pass and my identity card which is used to get access to various buildings. Starting the day I signed the forms, I am fully involved in the work in this program but only temporarily. Meanwhile, it was also very important that I make contact with the organization around our community providing employment services to job seekers.

Employment Ontario

One afternoon, I rang the office while at home. The person on the line quickly asked what the purpose of my calling was and what their office could do for me. I briefly stated that it was about your assistance for employment in agricultural fields I was looking. She said yes we can help you and requested that I just report to the office any time I am free with my identity documents showing I stay in Orleans. Any of the counsellors will see me on the first come first service basis. I went there and introduced myself to the secretary at the front desk. She recorded all my details including my needs, home and email addresses and the telephone numbers. Then she asked me to wait so that she could look for any available counsellor to attend to my problem. Employment Ontario is a service from the Ministry of Training, Colleges and Universities of Canada, which is handled by "La Cité collégiale" in Ontario, Canada. The institution helps job seekers and others in the province find work by providing various resources such as information about hiring companies, computers with internet access, fax machines, printers and telephones as well as personalized advice and services to help people assess their skills and experience, find work and start on the path to skills training. Other services they offer include individual counselling, résumé and interview preparation, job search techniques, career interest assessment, workshops and job fairs.

Few minutes later, I was called and introduced to one of the service counsellors. She took me to her cabinet and requested for additional personal details to use and open my file. After filling in the various forms, I was requested to read and sign them. Based on the information about my employment needs and career goals I provided, the counsellor concluded that I needed more individualized assistance and support that will help for the preparation of my "curriculum vitae" and for the search for an appropriate employment in my field of expertise. For this, she introduced me to another officer who will serve as my employment counsellor for my case. The first thing she indicated when we met was to have my certificates officially accessed to determine whether they could be accepted for employment in Canada.

Assessment of my credentials

The counsellor advised that one of the institutions which are well recognised by the government of Canada for evaluation of international academic achievements, confirmation of a degree obtained abroad and its eligibility for use for employment in Canada is World Education Services (WES) that can be found at the website http://www.wes.org/ca. The institution provides expert credential evaluations to immigrants to fulfill their employment in Canada so that one can pursue his or her professional career with confidence. She said Employment Ontario was going to pay the fees for assessment. During the next appointment day, she indicated it was apparent after consultation with her work mates that my degree from the United States will not have any problem for employment in Canada. Then, she indicated that the next priorities were to prepare a résumé for me both in French and English based on my CV, to write my teaching strategies and a template cover letter, and to identify potential employers who have recently advertised jobs in my field of expertise. It took us about 3 weeks, with meetings being arranged once a week due several other job seekers she had to attend to complete all necessary documents. When these were in place, I vigorously embarked on a computer searching for potential employers in agricultural fields including Canadian government agencies and university institutions mainly focussing on research and also on applying directly for jobs once an appropriate institution is found. During the searching, it become obvious that being member of the licencing body—Association of Agrologists—was among some of the most important conditions of employment in the agricultural field with my education qualification in Canada. I contacted some institutions to obtain conditions of eligibility to the Association to attain at least the Professional Agrologist status at P. Ag. level. Among the conditions were those of having a "graduate degree(s) in agricultural sciences or equivalent related discipline approved by the Admission and Registration Committee with 60 agrology credit hours or 20 full time courses from a recognized university." Moreover, I was again informed that the evaluation could be performed by WES and the final report be also sent to the Association of Agrologists.

For WES to initiate the evaluation process, it is requested for the interested individual to first register to provide details on the reasons for the assessment and to describe which type (s) of credential evaluation is needed. I provided all the information WES needed following my registration. Then, an account was open and the fees for the service I was looking for determined. I went back to Employment Ontario to discuss with the counsellor about the invoice and the possibility of them paying the fees on my behalf. It was agreed that I should pay and submit the receipt for reimbursement. I rapidly wrote and apply to Cornell University in US where I obtained my PhD degree in Plant Pathology requesting my transcripts. These were received three days later. I made copies together with those from my Master of Philosophy degree also in Plant Pathology from the University of Ibadan in Nigeria and the undergraduate degree ("Ingénieur Agronome") from the Faculty of Agriculture ("Institut Facultaire des Sciences Agronomiques á l'Université Nationale du Zaïre, now the Democratic Republic of Congo") which I mailed to WES. I wanted to establish whether these could be used to pursue my professional career in Canada and also if I had fulfilled the credit hours in agrology or the 20 full time courses with all my course credits from the various recognized universities I have attended to qualify for eligibility as a member of the Association of Agrologists in Canada.

First interview in Canada

It took nearly three months after several job applications went out that I received the first response for a telephone interview at a specified date and time early December 2013. This was for a position of Plant Pathologist for potato diseases. I read several documents related to the position some days before the interview and was ready for it. I was on stand-by near our telephone on the day and time which were indicated in the mail; but that call never came. I waited for nearly 15 minutes later and became anxious asking myself some questions whether I misread the mail. I quickly gone through the letter again because I had the print out with me, but realised that the date and the time were exactly as I had written down in my notebook. Five minutes went by, then ten minutes. I internally said to myself that maybe the interview has been called off without my knowledge. But, I also questioned that if it was cancelled why then they did not inform me. Nevertheless, I decided to wait for few more minutes and after about 15 minutes had elapsed in total, the telephone rang. I picked it rapidly and just heard one of the staff from their Human Resources apologising for the delay which was due to some technical problems. However, she said they were now ready for the proceeding. She explained that there were some Board members in the panel who will be asking some questions about different categories as per the work activities and also regarding overall management practices and interrelation with other workers. After the administrative explanation, one Board Member then provided additional information on the job description and requested if I had a question at this stage, which I did not have.

Thereafter, they immediately went on asking various questions such as those pertaining to my past work experience as it relates to the knowledge of potato diseases; my ability to communicate with several stakeholders particularly the growers and the industries with emphasis on providing specific examples during my carrier; giving clear instances where I had developed and implemented a program from the start to the end during my past field work; and whether the program was successful or not and explaining why. Additional questions concerned the capacity building of growers. Whether, in my past career, I have been involved in the training of stakeholders mainly farmers and extension agents and which tools were used for the training; If I am able to work without supervision from my highest authorities and how do I set priorities on multiple tasks and what strategies do I use to meet deadlines. Moreover, I had to describe any situation during my past career where my analytical approach to a given situation was incorrect and to illustrate briefly what I did to correct it. For this question I remained silent for a while looking for answer which could not come rapidly to my mind. I then asked the panel to proceed with other questions and return to it at a later stage since I could not immediately identify such situation. The panel continued by asking other questions such as how do I set regulations in crop protection; how could a specific pathogen for a given crop also affect weeds and how this is important for crop protection in general; whether I have any experience with the disease forecasting system; when am I available for the job if I am selected and finally, if I had any specific question for the board. Then, they returned to that question of providing an incorrect strategy to a situation to be solved and did I correct it. I simply indicated that I was unable to find a situation like that during my past work experience. Overall however, I answered the questions based on my past experience but often by referring to the situation at the institution. I also indicated that I was ready to start whenever I am notified to join the team and that I wanted to know more on the structure of my potential department to the question of availability and that of any question for the board, respectively. At this point they said the interview was completed and that candidates will be informed within 4 weeks. I thanked them and before hanging off the telephone the Human Resources again emphasized on some key elements concerning the conditions of employment including being allowed to work in Canada, having a valid driving license and being able to drive throughout various provinces of the country, and more importantly, If I was eligible for membership in the Institute of Agrologists. Only to this later I replied that I will have to inquire but that I was certain I am eligible for membership to the Canadian Phytopathological Society. By this time, I had already sent my credentials for evaluation at WES. Unfortunately a month later, I received a letter from the institution where I had interview that I was not successful for the position. Though I was disappointed, this could not discourage me from searching for employment to some additional institutions. I do not know where the next invitation for interview will come from. While waiting for that expected call, I enthusiastically and actively continue with my volunteer work at the Eastern Cereal and Oilseed Research Centre in Ottawa.

CHAPTER XIV

MY HEALTH SUPPORT

*T*he journey through my sickness has been full of hardship particularly from the various treatments and related side effects, and the acute pain I considerably endured both prior to the sickness diagnosis and during the hospitalization and medical follow-ups at home. Managing such a painful situation could not

I was so lucky to have received support from many people and different institutions including my family members and friends. Their compassion went a long way in the healing process and caring during the journey of my sickness.

have been possible without the assistance from various sources. There have been on the course of the sickness several occasions during which I experienced acute and intolerable pain, and almost an unmanageable loss of energy and appetite always leading to dramatic weight loss. During such periods, I was often unable to speak and only barely open eyes or walk necessitating the presence of others to take care of my various needs. As it has been well documented (Amgen Canada Inc., 2010), many people generally become compassionate for cancer patients to the point of fully providing their hands to support and care about their multitude concerns. I was so lucky to receive assistance from different people and institutions including my family members, relatives and friends. Their compassion went a long way as an important part of the healing and caring in the journey of my sickness.

Family support

The first thing I did upon my arrival in Canada was to speak with my spouse and the children about the various events in my sickness. As I continued talking to them, I realized that they all became concerned about my health status and how thin I was as compared to my normal look and body weight they knew. They were in presence of a complete different person this time. Amazingly, the sickness rapidly recreated our family intimacy and warmth relationship becoming the unifying building block around which my spouse and all the children (Fig. 25) regularly gathered. I have been separated from them for almost five years when they came to Canada and I remained in Zambia. Indeed, I received the LORD's grace through the compassion of my nearby relatives. I was surprised to see that all of them turned the focus of their attention to a sound consolation and most care I so needed. Their solid attachment to me during this journey has since become unforgettable particularly because all were so moved by the sickness to the point of giving up their precious daily undertakings to concentrate on my care. Talking regularly to them or seeing them constantly around me either in the hospital or at home made us closer, considerably reducing the persistent stress and anxiety I was enduring, and restoring my peace, rejoicing my heart and more importantly acting as a major source of the disease healing.

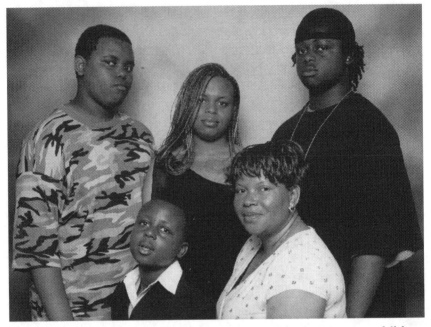

Figure 25. From left to the right and top to the bottom my children Jonathan Kadyma, Divine Muimba, Dereck Kabeya, Emmanuel Muimba and my spouse Ngabwa-Kabeya

In addition to her full time work, my spouse Ngabwa-Kabeya always stood by me throughout the journey of my sickness. We have been married since 1984 without any previous dating period and we are still together without any major family dispute. Although from time to time we encounter some problems that could lead to a strong opposition of ideas, we always found a terrain of reconciliation that keeps us unified. The first day I met her at one of my friends' home, who happened to be her sister's husband, signs of togetherness suddenly developed between us. The attraction between us became spontaneous. Since then, I strongly felt I have met the lovely companion I dearly wanted for so long in my life and a friend I could share my innermost secrets with. A close woman I could talk to about the intimacy from my heart. I loved her look and more importantly how soft she was talking to me. After few months, we finally committed to joyfully become a couple and form a family. Starting the time when she realized the poor conditions in which I was when I reached Canada from Africa, she instantly decided—on the family's behalf—to have the hospital take directly care of my health. The best memory I have is when she urgently called the ambulance, on two occasions based on her own judgement, to dispatch me rapidly to the emergency department in the hospital considering the seriousness of my situation. Additionally, she had been always reminding me in every single day about the date and the time for the next appointment, making sure I was fully committed to all the follow up consultations with medical staff, provision of blood and/or urine for laboratory analyses and the other numerous tests required for my health.

To this moment when I am about to complete the writing of this book, I have gone through four major surgeries after more than 132 consultations with medical doctors, according to my diary, and about 45 to 50 laboratory analyses and radiological tests. Under the appointment records in my diary, I had clearly indicated the date, time, and the person I was going to meet and at which place as well as the purpose of the appointment such as the treatment types and kind of the test to be carry out. This chart was looked at daily before going to bed to ensure I am always ready with the hospital visits. Some other tests are still requested by doctors each 6 months for the next 5 years to assess whether the cancer has been completely eradicated or has reoccurred. During treatments, my spouse was my driver to and from the hospital and to other several places where I needed to go for any medical attention. There were also some intermittent helps of my driving by the children. However, more important have been times when she lifted and walked me to either the bathroom or the toilet when I lacked energy to do it by myself, and bathed, put lotion and dressed me when I was unable to do so. She prepared meal for me and brought it in the bed where I was laying, most of the time, without force to reach the dining table, and constantly did my laundry to avoid unclean clothing from blood stains, urine leak, stool accidently discharged and unforeseen germs that might contaminate me and other family members after a long stay in the hospital setting. She always prayed for my circumstances and constantly pleaded for my healing to Almighty, Jehovah the LORD in heaven.

My children are now all grown up with the first of the five, a girl, being 29 years old and the last, a boy, 16 years old. There is a universal say stipulating that *"Children are true gift from God."* In line with this, Bonnke (2004) also wrote *"God places an immense value on earthy kinships, from one generation to another."* Furthermore, he gave biblical illustrations referring to family ties between the farther, the mother and the children and specifically highlighted numerous scripture passages in the bible in which reference is made to matter regarding the family. Generally, children feel indebted to parents for what they have gained over time and what they have become at moment. In the Bantu Luba culture and system—an ethnic and a sub-tribe group in the eastern Kasai Province in DR Congo where my family originates—the family is often organized through kinship groups. Its structure is characterized by membership to patrilineal clans (descent through males) in which one another help ensures the social cohesion. In this system, the family is the unit of one's life and consists of the life of each man with his descendants. Although it generally encompasses his wife or several women at times up to three or four as wives and the siblings, a single family will always be composed of a large group of related people which may include of the extended family such as other relatives living within the same household including brothers, sisters, parents, cousins, nieces, nephews, uncles, aunts, grandparents. The father is the household's head, the provider of the family's needs and the leader of the family that is formed around certain rules, attributes, tasks, habits and beliefs etc. Children are always expected to be obedient and respectful of elders often listen to adult while facing down. They are supposed to receive anything given to them with their two hands and then reply in return "thank you." They have specific endless responsibilities vis-à-vis their parents inherent not only from the clan and passed from generation to generation but also from God. For instance, it is well illustrated in [EXODUS 20: 12] how the LORD set a clear commandment for the children that:

"Honour your father and your mother, so that you may live long in the land the LORD your God is giving you..."

This same command is also well recognized as part of the children's rights to parents in the moral civic of my country. It may also be so for some other countries. Among the most important and valuable gifts they provide to parents are warmth love and care, but children often also offer other assistance to parents ranging from food, clothes, home to live in and financial resources depending on their possibilities. This culture, which is deeply rooted in our original traditional culture, always necessitates for collective solidarity and reciprocity. In this way, each other assistance is current whereby collective services and additional items are shared among members of the community when one is in need. We eat together sharing one plate often using our hands around fire in the evening and also share our labor force for any work such as building a house or ploughing the field.

As far as my family is concerned, I did not initially know how my children's reaction could be after learning that the farther had cancer. I had considerable fear that they might just consider this as any simple sickness that one could be infected with and hence, they might just continue the course of their life without caring for me. More so, I was greatly afraid that my sickness would probably modify our relationship with the children especially considering that the sickness had significantly reduced my working capability to provide for them, now relying only on their mother's performance of the various tasks both at workplace and at home for the provision of the household's needs. I was really worrying about my life, but also I acknowledged this was a new encounter for me and accepted to live with. There was no any other choice for life than going through it and vigorously fight against it. In the contrary and to my surprise, the sickness made our relationships even grow stronger bringing them closer to me and all becoming very much caring, loving and sympathetic with my new health status. I was so shocked to read on their face when I finished explaining and sharing with them that very sad information about the onset of the symptoms and signs of the disease as well as its final diagnosis. Though I could read a painful emotion and the expression of sadness on their face when I finally said I have been found with cancer, they all however immediately accepted the situation. I knew this because of the fact that the youngest and the third boys suddenly hugged me and said "Oh! Daddy, we love you." Those staying with us at home constantly helped as they could despite their school endeavor whereas those already living out our house continued asking many questions particularly how I was feeling any time they gathered around me as family or through telephone conversation and email system. Such compassion, they all expressed, considerably restored my strength.

The two vehicles belonging to the first and the third children, respectively, were sometimes also used to carry me for appointments to the hospital whenever our own vehicle was with the mother at work or had some mechanical problem. When I was urgently taken to the emergency department in the ambulance as a result of colostomy prolapse leading to a portion of the intestine coming out of the abdomen, they made sure one of their siblings was behind it to know at which hospital I was taken to. They regularly also visited either one by one or as a group in the hospital to comfort me. During such visits, they often brought numerous items such as fruits, juices and reading material that will help keeping me busy. In addition, my daughter brought her laptop computer I could use to check my mails or listen to music on the CDs when I had strength. The fourth boy went even further by cancelling to proceed with his academic education for a year after graduation from the secondary program or to find a job which could procure money for him and decided just to remain with me at home when everybody was out. During annual events such as Christmas, Easter, Father Days and others, they always decorated home, brought presents and stayed around for long time to entertain and distract me from the stress and anxiety. In certain occasions, they also took me outdoor for a walk to stretch out my body knowing that walking, as a physical activity, will significantly improve someone's health by strengthening bones and lifting the mood and through the prevention of such unhealthy conditions like the heart disease, high blood pressure and diabetes.

Not only talking regularly to the children gave me hope for living but also this became my major source of the mind healing and long life. At times also, I received their feeling and reaction to my illness. One day, my youngest had pointed out that "Dad, you are very thin as compared to your weight before." Similarly, all the boys often wondered "when will the pouch in the abdomen be removed?" Such questions, although upsetting and frustrating, always reminded me they were very much concerned about me and wanted that I return rapidly back to my normal situation they were familiar with than I could by myself. Listening to this reaction often triggered in me a guilty feeling about what they were facing as a result of my sickness. However, I always thanked them and sincerely appreciated for any help they were providing. I also tried, as much as I could, to encourage them to persevere with what they are doing but also forcibly not to show I was in acute pain to avoid raising a number of questions of concern in their mind about my future life. Rather, I always showed a very positive attitude towards my current situation. In this way, I ensured them I was strong and confident although in extensive distress.

Beside the close members of family, my spouse's and owns siblings also played another key role in my comfort during the sickness period. Those outside Canada constantly called to know how I was doing or find out about the progress on the various treatments I was getting for the sickness and to also wish me a rapid health recovery. Their concern about the cancer that has affected my health was overwhelming. They often encouraged me for persistence over the treatments to conquer the disease. Similarly, not only those staying in Canada—who are my spouse's two sisters living in Gatineau in Quebec Province and Galgary in Alberta Province—called almost every day but they also frequently visited either at home or when I was admitted in the hospital to comfort me and bring their morale support.

Friends' support

Having friends around and being connected to so many of them worldwide was as the best and important key of hope for my health recovery, working indeed as a strong medication that has been prescribed to cure the diagnosed cancer. When they got news that I was very sick with cancer in Canada, both old and new friends amazingly made contact with us either on telephone, using on-line facilities or through a post card to show their attachment and provided morale support during this hard time my family and I were going through. It was not easy for me, but I never felt lonely or I was not like one who is undergoing severe experience of distress because I was always with a view that friends were still around me although being at very distant places. Some of them, particularly those from the United States beside writing letters, they organized themselves for a group to visit me in Canada at the time when I was under chemotherapy treatment and very sick. Apparently, they circulated the news of my sickness among several students as well as to faculty members in the various university departments I attended in US. Before the team which included my PhD supervisor during my graduate studies in US and some classmates with whom we had formed a research group to discuss scientific issues of interest under the leadership of my supervisor arrived, my inbox email was filled with messages wishing me a "Get Well Muimba." They came to show their moral support and amazingly, they also brought their financial support. Receiving them physically at our home after several years we separated following my return to Africa made me feel new and bright although I was still very weak with the chemotherapy treatment. Sitting and discussing together around the table created in my innermost a wealth of warmth. They are so wonderful in my heart. Sincerely, I feel lucky coming across such great friends in my life.

While on graduate studies at Cornell University in the United States between 1987 and 1991, I never felt lonely or had severe experience of homesickness. It happened that my Department in particular and the University in general were home to a very multi-racial population of both undergraduate and graduate students. Nevertheless, being away from older friends and other family members in Africa for a long time; living in an unfamiliar environment and meeting new people; and mostly struggling with a different and harsh climate prevailing in the Northeastern part of the States were not always easy at least for the initial periods of my study. The culminating effect of all these conditions quickly preconditioned my body to high stress levels and culture shock. It took, however, a very short time that I completed my adjustment to become fully part of the general American society and the university surroundings. I rapidly became acquainted with several places within the location to find whatever items I needed including many people to speak to about any of my concern. I met friends both in the department I was registered and others as well. More importantly capitalizing on the great sense of togetherness existing within the research group under the leadership of Professor Gary Bergstrom, today my mentor; I created what I qualify as my lifetime great friendships with fellow American classmates as well as students from other continents with whom I continue being in close contact up to this time.

Everyone in the group was keen to know other colleague's progress in their study and always provided constructive scientific advice for improvement to others' research. During group meetings, topics for discussion were always stimulating and enlightening. Some of the most valuable close, heartedly and great friends I made at Cornell include Gary Bergstrom's family, Rowe Neil Miller's family, Nancy Keller, Schilder Annemick, Christine Stockwell, Diane Florini's family, David Yohalen, Denis A. Shah, Kent Loeffler and Dave Kalb to name but a few. I was privileged to have wonderful graduate students like Nancy Keller and Diana Florini for their valuable advice and directions. They helped me immeasurably from the accommodation-hunting, setting up utilities and bank accounts and so on, to the more ephemeral things like learning US body language and speech conventions. I will never also forget David H. Thurston, a very encouraging faculty member, who tirelessly spent most of his time providing endless advice for continuous perseverance in my endeavor as well as other faculty including William Fry, Tom A. Zitter, Jim Lobeer, Gillian Turgeon, Steve Beer, Alan Collmer, George Hudler and Margaret Smith for their continuous support to date.

Another wonderful family I became acquainted to in US is the Stella Coakley's family. I came across this family while in Boulder, Colorado, for the preparation of the English proficiency prior to my graduate study at Cornell. Stella Coakley is also a Phytopathologist as I am whereas her husband, Jim Coakley, is a Geophysicist. All the children, at the time when I was introduced to the Coakley's, were within their youngest age. They rapidly became closer to me and being always by my side any time I visited their home. Now Martha, Sarah and Mirian are adults and have their own families. Over since, the Coakley's family has been at my heart all the time and we have remained in touch constantly sharing news about our respective families. When I shared with them information on my sickness, I was delighted to read from their numerous mails how shocked and affected they became. They were compassionate and always there for me regardless of this devastating disease. They sent several post-cards and the family journal with lovely words of comfort from the bottom of their hearts wishing for all the best in my health recovery. Indeed, several of such friendships I made in US have lasted forever, and even widely open up for me more opportunities for a global working network in the field of plant protection.

Similarly few weeks later, we were again fortunate to have another visit by another friend's family, the Mahungu Zola Meso's, but this time from the DR Congo (Fig. 26). Mahungu's spouse had come to Canada to visit the children who are settled in Montreal,

Quebec, for some family matters. Since she was aware of my sickness, the opportunity of her presence in the country was taken to stop by our home to express their concern and comfort to me. We graduated for the Bachelor degree in agriculture from the Faculty of Agriculture at the National University of DR Congo, then Zaïre, the same year with Mahungu. Thereafter, we were together offered a job in the Ministry of Agriculture for a project to improve cassava production (PRONAM) in Bas-Congo before we joined the International Institute for Tropical Agriculture (IITA) as Regional Agronomists. Later, Mahungu became the Coordinator of another IITA project (SARRNET) in Malawi in Southern Africa and later the Country's Representative for IITA in DR Congo. Mahungu and other old close workmates just after graduation for Bachelor degree in agriculture including Muaka Toko currently a

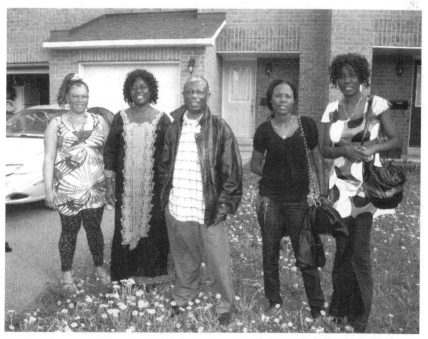

Figure 26. A family friend from the Democratic Republic of Congo in visit to Montreal stopped at our house in Orleans to know about my health status

research scientist in the Republic of Benin and Kiala Kilusi Ngudi Wa Se, a Professor at Agostino Neto University in Angola, have kept our friendship tight since our first meeting in 1972. We regularly communicate on family issues as well as other matters concerning our life and the future.

Several other friends throughout Ottawa in Canada particularly those in our neighbourhood in Orleans also paid visit to discuss my health issues and to comfort me. During the discussion, I always openly and honestly shared the cancer problem and my feeling over it with them so they could understand what I was going through and how I was concentrating all my effort to mitigate it. Often, they enquired on what have been medical doctors' views about the sickness and whether there were still some more treatments that I needed to take to eradicate the disease. Additionally, they always tended to keep me busy with laughter talks often checking on my reaction to their jokes. I considered this as a relaxation therapy for a relief from on-going stress, unhappiness and anxiety I was enduring. Similarly, they persistently wanted to know how they could be of further help including the possibility of taking me to the hospital and provision of foods. But also, they always provided for their emotional support and wished me to get well from the sickness. I found their moral support useful in building up my positive attitude which is necessary in the strengthening and comforting my self being regardless of the situation I was in. Talking and laughing together often made my life more fulfilling and our relationship more loving.

Support from the hospital administration

Clinical managers and several other staff from the hospital administration also provided significant additional care which I enormously needed during hospitalization and home care. They visited at certain occasions to check on me and promptly responded to my call whenever I was looking for something of urgent concern. The meal from the hospital was always given on time; my inpatient room repeatedly cleaned and bed sheets regularly changed to ensure standard sanitation around the patient. All relevant information regarding the various treatments I was subjected to for cancer control was thoroughly explained to me and well detailed to my spouse when I was unable to follow the explanation due to the acute pain. Related pamphlets and booklets were also provided.

However, I recall one single instance when I was very much furious, upset and frustrated about one particular nurse. This was during one evening when I was in serious discomfort crying because of severe pain after the surgery and insertion of the nephrostomy. The pain was so agonizing and out of proportion that I rang the bell calling for assistance. I could not sleep. I was completely exhausted with no energy to do anything like moving out of bed or walking. One of my attending nurses for that night shift reported to the room. She found me weeping and uncomfortably rolling on the bed due to the severe pain. Then, she asked:

"How can I help you?"
"I am in severe pain and cannot leave the bed to go to the toilet to clean up the ostomy push which is nearly full," I responded.
"Sorry sir, I cannot help you. You need to make an effort and do it by yourself in the toilet which is close to you." She said.
"I am unable to do it please, please." I screamed.
"Sorry dear, I cannot help you." she insisted that I should try to get out of the bed and go to the toilet.
"Is there any other nurse who can assist me please?" I repeatedly and loudly screamed for I became so nervous.
"I am the one designated for care in this room." She pointed out to me.

I waited for so long still screaming but realized that no one else came to my rescue. I slowly forced myself with that severe pain—just as she had requested and I will not forget this—to leave the bed and reach the toilet to clean out the stool in the ostomy pouch. At that point I decided in my mind to report the nurse's unfriendly behavior to the next nurse or the hospital management. After considerable thoughts on the issue throughout the night as I could not sleep well and the following morning, I came to a conclusion that maybe she was right. I said to myself maybe she acted so on my own best interest to learn how to manage the ostomy regardless of the discomfort. Maybe! After sometimes, I reached the conclusion that I should not take the case any further. Otherwise however, I was constantly taken care of during all periods of my hospitalization in any of the Ottawa hospitals. Of a very particular importance to point out has been the spiritual care from the hospital chaplain. During the visit, the chaplain asked various questions about the sickness and my family, and always listened carefully to my story. I am surely convinced this was so for other patients. Some of the things I was relating were always about my constant fear of cancer that has caused death of many people, the confusion I was going through in my mind, the acute pain I was regularly experiencing, my prolonged isolation while in the hospital, the depression and hopelessness I was feeling mainly due to loss of income now relying only on my spouse to meet our household needs. The Chaplain's visit and advice always brought hope, encouragement for healing and a sense of not being lonesome. It considerably enlisted me with joyfulness and strength to face again vigorously the various aspects of my sickness life—physical, mental, emotional and relational—without fear but with hope.

Home care support

Following every discharge from any of the hospitals where I have been admitted and considering that the period of hospitalization has always been very short often lasting between three to seven days before being released, an arrangement was always made through the Community Care Access Center (CCAC, http://www.

champlainccac-ont.ca) for follow up home care services. CCAC staff and the hospital always planned for the patient's discharge taking into consideration the amount and type of home care he/she will need while at home after leaving the hospital. Before leaving the hospital, a CCAC representative has always visited my room to let me know about arrangements for home care services once I am discharged. As it is in CCAC's policies, the Center will designate the patient's Care Manager/Care Coordinator whose responsibilities are to develop the patient's care plan according to the various health issues at hand and following the recommendations from the hospital. Moreover, it always ensured that the patient is provided with quality and professional healthcare services that meet his or her needs. After assessing my health needs, the Coordinator subcontracted another professional healthcare organization for the delivery—at home—of the nursing services needed often based on mutual trust, respect and understanding. For this, CCAC required that members of my family and I become full participants in the healthcare package being provided. This was achieved through the administration of a series of questions related to my health history and the overall family's background. The family is also required to raise any questions when something is unclear or of concern such as any practice by nurses in unhealthy or unprofessional ways. Indeed on my discharge days, the hospital had requested the CCAC to take up with the nursing home care for the stoma, the colostomy and ileostomy, the surgery wounds, radiation and chemotherapy treatments as well as related effects, nephrostomy and stent implants. The institution had also an eye on matters regarding several other issues related to my health such as procurement of needed supplies and medications.

Carefor

Carefor Health and Community Services, I will refer to in the book as Carfor (http://www.carefor.ca), provided for most of my home nursing care during this illness journey. This is one of the charitable organizations offering home health care appropriate to patient needs and community support services in Ottawa and some surrounding counties. The support includes care for retired seniors' residents, programs for homeless and mental clinics, meal services, transportation programs and nursing for palliative care as well as health and wellness clinics. The request the organization put forward prior to its nurses' visits at home was for members of my household to refrain from indoor smoking and wearing scents. Moreover, we had to notify the office in case we had pets such as dogs so let nurses be aware of this. In such case, we had to isolate the pets in other rooms whenever nurses were visiting. Fortunately, none of the above applied to our home.

The first day the Carefor nurse visited was after my discharge from the civic hospital following the colostomy surgery. The service the nurse provided consisted basically of my training about the "Fall Risk Assessment for Patients with Pre-disposing Medical Conditions." She evaluated my health conditions based on 10-risk factors ranging from age and mental status to sensory deficits and current daily medication intake. Then, I was given necessary information on my role during home care services— have the right to participate in own care by asking questions for clarification when something was unclear; should be treated with respect and dignity; be able to say yes or no to the service being offered; I should be ensured of the privacy and confidentiality of my medical information; and voice concerns or complaints to the organization management any time I felt my privacy has been compromised. My responsibility as well as that of my family members was to treat the visiting nurses and other staffs from the organization with courtesy and respect; notify the office at least 24 hours in advance whenever I was unavailable for home visit; keep the health charts in a safe place and return these at the completion of the services; and fully collaborate with the organization to facilitate its meeting of the established health care goals. Nurses' rights and responsibilities were also briefed, mainly consisting of following standard nursing procedures for home care and recording all aspects of the services given to the patient.

For care of the surgery wound after it had ruptured and the ostomy, Carefor nurses assisted first with an intensive coaching on how to get out of the bed and climbing stairs. Thereafter, they daily removed old dressings, aseptically cleaned on the wound and stoma areas and covered the cleaned site with new patches of sterile dressing packs. Each time, the size of the wound and the percentage of tissue recovery as well as the nature and amount of exudation from the wound and the stoma, the rate of healing, and the pain endured and discomfort felt were monitored and recorded. The characteristics for the stoma and types of appliances used to cover it including their source were also recorded. Any allergic reaction observed onto the surface around the stoma was also reported and managed accordingly using appropriate interventions to curtail the rush. During the times I was very weak as a result of the radiation and chemotherapy treatments, pain from surgeries and wound infection, and when I had nausea as well as continuous difficulty with my respiration particularly during night times, they often flushed out and wiped the pouch and sealed it back, and provided medications allowing sleeping well. Similarly, they flushed out the PICC and nephrostomy lines and redressed them with fresh moisture resistant barrier always ensuring the lines had not migrated far out from the initial point where they were initially inserted. To ensure lines were perfectly working, nurses checked for an easy flow of the flashing fluid and the blood's return. Any blood drainage in the nephrostomy tube into bag was rapidly reported to the appropriate medical doctor for further assessment and alternative courses of action to take. Due to recurrent germ infection my system was subjected to, nurses always also disconnected the chemotherapy tubing, and flushed and closed its opening in readiness for the next infusion after microbial treatment. Of particular concern to nurses during the visits were also my low appetite, the constant bad mood and a persistent feeling of nausea resulting particularly from the chemotherapy treatment. In such conditions, they always ensured I took a large quantity of fluids such as juice with flavor, at least 1-2 L each day. They also continued with the provision of medications as prescribed by the hospital at the discharge times and the disposition of used needles and syringes in appropriate disposable containers.

At the end of a chemotherapy treatment cycle, they discontinued the PICC line flushing but also removed the lining as requested by the hospital. It became commonly obvious that my arm skin at the site where the PICC line was inserted constantly developed severe itchy rushes. They treated these by applying an antibiotic-medicated powder each day. At the same time, they continued with monitoring and handling of the surgery wound and ostomy care while also training me for ostomy—the flange and the bag—handling mainly the discharge of the stool, the cleaning and rinsing, and for the replacement with and the closing of a new pouch. Similarly, they regularly handled the cleaning of the nephrostomy tube and the area around the insertion site during the time I had this catheter to prevent urinary tract infection and skin breakdown and made observation of the urine color as well as possible occurrence of sediment in it. As days advanced, I became independent for the stoma and flange management and care. Generally, Carefor through CCAC provided initial ostomy supplies and ordered several other needed medical items for my home care at the Ontario Medical Supplies (OMS). However, more additional supplies throughout the period of bowel resting and healing were obtained using funds from a grant I received from the Assistive Devices Program (ADP) by the Canadian Ministry of Health and Long-Term Care. This was after submitting hospital forms I signed together with the surgeon. However, costs for other several drugs and ambulance to the emergency department were incurred by my family. Carefor nurses also regularly assessed my health status and rapidly reported their findings to the hospital especially when there was development of an unusual abnormal condition. In regard of this, it was the Carefor nurse, whom my family had called the night when the VAC pump was saturated with blood and a mucus-like infected fluid from the wound, who rapidly sent me back to the hospital emergency department. She reported home within a short time and on her assessment of the situation, she immediately called 911 for an ambulance to take me to the hospital. My family and I sincerely thank Carefor for the professionalism, commitment, enthusiasm and tirelessly work of its nursing staff for my health during the entire period of my sickness. You attended to me just on time during the peak of my sickness when the vital care was needed, and I am certainly convinced that your hands have been the main key to my surgery wound healing and my health recovery.

Bayshore Home Health Care

As for Carefor, the Bayshore health care (http://www.bayshore.ca) is also among the home and community health care providers in Ottawa. The organization offers a multitude of nursing services including personal and home support care. It was also sub-contracted by CCAC to handle home care for my surgery wound following the reversal of the ileostomy to the natural anus at the General Hospital. Immediately after I was discharged, after a week of hospitalization, Bayshore was contacted for follow up care services at home. Nurses from Bayshore visited the same day in the evening when I was home for the initial contact, to assess my health status and provide the provisional time table for visits. The following days and onwards, they performed the various duties as those earlier achieved by Carefor nurses. They mainly included maintaining post-surgical wound by changing dressings, pain and symptom management, and provision of medications as prescribed by the hospital. More importantly however, they had a crucial task of regularly pulling out and filling in the opening that was left in the middle of the wound during the surgery with sterile gauze. After the old gauze was removed, nurses aseptically wiped out the abdominal area around the wound, monitored the wound depth and width by recording the measures to establish its healing progress and then covered it with fresh sterile packing and dressings. In this process, they closely followed the midline abdominal incision the surgeon had mad during the surgery, packed it with normal saline-soaked 0.6 cm x 4.6 m Curity™ Plain

Packing Gauze Strip and applied tegaderm foam to certainly ensure its protection from any external possible infection. After about a month and half, staples that served to suture the wound were removed without major problems, and the wound healing process continued normally. By exactly two months after I left the hospital, the wound was completely closed without any incident and healed remarkably well. At this time, nurses decided to stop covering it with the dressings. Personally as a patient, this open wound surface became of concern. I requested that they continue covering it for a while for sanitary safety. They trained to do it by myself since it had already reached a good healing stage which was not of concern for them. I managed the wound surface by protecting it with sterile dressings for nearly about additional two weeks when I stopped. The area that was incised had completed sealed off. As for Carefor, they also professionally handled the surgery wound as well as other health issues I encountered from the day I was discharged from the hospital to its healing. They remain at my heart for the diligent services they performed and valuable support at the time I was sick.

Support from volunteers

Many volunteers operate in the various hospital departments mainly to guide, help and assist patients and their families for any needs they may want. In my case, volunteers were instrumental to my health right from the beginning of my cancer diagnosis and treatment. Using their own first-hand experience, they also trained me about all the clinical procedures I will be expecting during my treatments, toured the participating team of patients to the various facilities in the hospital Cancer Center, and provided initial important training and reading resources (e.g. brochures) to better understanding the cancer disease and how it can be handled. Similarly, they distributed relevant information about available community-based services and resources that would be of immensurable assistance to patients as they embark on their journey to cancer treatments. On several occasions the volunteers were also helpful in providing directions to various sites of appointments in the hospital and often visited in the ward room to chat and bring comfort as well. Voluntarism among Canadians has considerably astonished me. Having people sharing their time with other unknown people without anything in return is generally not common in Africa, except in the context of community belonging I had earlier explained. One will help other relatives often with the sense of community sustenance and continuity. Otherwise however, the assistance from volunteers was also primordial to my health recovery and this should be used by any other patients.

CHAPTER XV

CONCLUSION

While at my workplace at the Copperbelt University in Zambia, I began to have a generalised body malaise, suffering from an unknown sickness. This resulted in a considerable health deterioration characterized by a sudden weight loss, a continuous rising of the blood pressure, anemia, weakness, tiredness and dizziness, and more importantly a rectal bleeding each time I was in the toilet for stool discharge. All these abnormal syndromes made it difficult to efficiently perform my work. Following a visit at a local clinic, a rectal tumor—measuring about 110 x 81 mm size—was observed and recommendations were suggested for its urgent removal through a surgical operation. I was shocked and frightened to hear this news of a tumor in my body. I suddenly began panicking and becoming nervous and sad, not believing about it although the finding did not establish whether the tumor was cancerous. That day was the darkest moment I ever known in my life. As devastated as I was, I informed my family in Canada about the tumor and the recommendations from the local hospital. They rapidly arranged for me to travel to Canada and the same day I arrived, I was rushed to the General Hospital in Ottawa where a stage III to IV colorectal cancer was finally diagnosed following several specialized laboratory tests and analyses.

To tackle the sickness, I was first subjected to an urgent surgery to bypass a portion of the colon that was obstructed by the tumor to allow for the bowel discharge through an external artificial pouch appliance on the stoma. Then, I went through an adjuvant chemo-radiation therapy to shrink the tumor considering its large size for an immediate surgery to remove it. During the course of the radiation and chemotherapy treatments, I experienced numerous side effects the main ones being nausea and some vomiting; minimal loss of appetite mostly due to dry mouth as well as the development of some sore in the mouth making the food tasteless than usual; partial hair loss; body itching mainly in the eyes; tingling of the hand palms and feet soles; loss of sensation to touch particularly when it is cold; skin burning becoming darkish particularly on the face and the arm around the area where the chemotherapy drugs were infused; general fatigue often feeling very tired and weak; and numbness in the toes and feet. My body was indeed like being mutilated.

Following treatments, the tumor was removed in a 9-hour surgery after which I developed several other setbacks. The most important and worrisome among these were the recurrent microbial infection and continuous surgery wound infection and the kidney failure as well. As a result, the wound from surgery to remove the tumor took about 7 months to heal. To speed up the healing process during this time, the wound site was connected to a vacuum pump to facilitate the suction of discharged mucus-like infected fluid via a tube into a canister. In this way, the pump would work as a negative pressure therapy pulling together the cells around the wound to accelerate the healing. Instead of drawing the infected fluid, the pump unfortunately sucked a large amount of my blood leading to anemia, pale skin and nearly my death. I was urgently transfused with 5 units of blood, inserted with a stent and nephrostomy to allow free flow of urine from the ureter to the bladder because of kidney dysfunction and readmitted in the hospital for a long period.

During hospitalization, I faced the shadow of death as a result of acute pain, not eating and general body discomfort and illness resulting in considerable weight loss. Because I was so desperate for the relief and quick alleviation of the problem of the acute pain I was enduring, any medication that could help in this situation was just welcomed. Fortunately, I have been so lucky to have a good quality and highest standard healthcare at the hospital and at home in Ottawa. Medical doctors and residents as well as nurses worked tirelessly and with commitment to promptly attend to my numerous health problems. Nevertheless, visions of death were always rooming around through the death dreams and nightmares. My spouse and I rapidly understood this sickness was more of spiritual than physical battle that we needed to fully rely on the LORD and trust Him to overcome it. As such, we solemnly declared the healing victory just as David said when he faced the giant and powerful giant Goliath [SAMUEL 17: 1-58]. My battling with cancer was already won through the LORD Jesus Christ. I thanked and praised Him every morning when I wake up and every night before going to bed for I am in good health without any sickness today. My faith for God's healing considerably increased through reading the Bible as well as other Christian magazines, and through personal's, families', friends' and pastors' prayers. I surely know and I am certain that He made possible the trip to Lubumbashi in DR Congo for the initial statement on the sickness and to Canada for its conclusive diagnosis. There is always no victory without carrying the cross. He took me through a harsh and very difficult journey of medical procedures and side effects that I endured to the Healing and Health Recovery. "Thank you JESUS".

I went again through another very long postoperative cycle of chemotherapy regimen to kill the possible remnant cancerous cells adjacent to the tumor and undertook various tests, particularly the CEA and CT scan of the abdomen and pelvis, as requested by Oncologists to ascertain a complete eradication of the sickness. Test results following the treatment and 6 months later were all negative showing no signs of cancer. I praised the LORD for the healing. In a similar way by His grace, the ileostomy was reversed and the colon reconstructed to allow for bowel movement and stool discharge from the natural anus. Because of the weakness of the sphincter muscle necessary for continence regulation, stool continually ran without restrain considering that this muscle at the anal peripheral has not been working for the last two or so years. Its perineal strengthening exercises were then regularly performed to improve its full recovery to a satisfactory level to provide for the pelvic floor strength that could defer bowel movement further when walking around, sleeping or in a meeting etc. Glory be to the Heavenly Majesty that this muscle is slowly reaching its initial status.

To ensure the 6-month period results were conclusively consistent with those from the previous tests just after the chemotherapy treatment, Oncologists requested that I took further tests including the positron emission tomography (PET) scan. They stated that "this test is very expensive and they are not always allowed to recommend it for patients." PET scan uses some radiation to make detailed pictures of the body parts, therefore showing how well the chemistry of the various organs and other tissues function or could be affected by cancer. Consistently, all results were negative with no signs of cancer recurrence. Moreover, a further colonoscopy test was requested by the surgeon to check on the full colon conduit, and it revealed a well healed colon.

The course of this colorectal cancer that was diagnosed in my body has been full of hardship and suffering. There have been times when I could not speak, open eyes or walk, being in general discomfort necessitating others to assist and care for my various needs. During some of such circumstances, I managed to sit by the window in my patient ward room so that I could at least watch outside as some of the rooms had a good external view. I continued observing vehicles passing and also contemplating how people were actively moving in all directions. I felt hopelessness. But, I was still faithful to my LORD for the healing. I should confidently confess and loudly vouch that this was certainly the most enriching experience in my life. I was blessed to have support from various sources such as my spouse and children, close relatives, friends, both doctors and hospital and home care nurses, and various volunteers who were compassionate and helpful. I received nothing but an immense support from all of them. Their close relationships, friendships and passionate care all went a long way as an important tool for a considerable reduction of my stress and anxiety, therefore restoring my peace, rejoicing and comforting my heart, and more importantly acting as a major source of my healing. Friends who had previously experienced the similar illness in their family opened up to me about their own case, or that of people they knew and loved. I considerably learnt how to cope with cancer from them.

I thereby openly say to all of you that you have eternally remained at the center of my heart and in the fore of my mind for the kindness help on my behalf. Moreover, the several hours I spent at the Ottawa Cancer Foundation and to other community or social services were as well fruitful in learning how to adjust my lifestyle post-cancer treatments. Out of my sickness, I have learnt many things that have now made me better prepared than ever before, and more awaken and realistic about cancer.

Thank you Lord for what You have done for me

Bibliography

1) About Cancer: Overview. Cancer Research UK. (2005, 03/11). CancerHelp UK. Birmingham, UK: Cancer Research UK.

2) Barbour Publishing Inc., 2007. 199 Promises of God. Uhrichsville, Ohio. USA.

3) Amgen Canada Inc., 2010. Colorectal Cancer and You: A Guide for People Living with Colorectal Cancer 2nd ed. Colorectal Cancer Association of Canada. Toronto, Canada. 53pp.

4) Billett, B., 2008. Praying With Fire: Praying Effectively Using God's Word! Zondervan Co. Grand Rapids, Michigan. USA. 103pp.

5) Bonnke, R., 2004. Winning Your Friends and Family to Christ. Full Flame, LLC. Florida, USA. 28pp.

6) Bressa, G.L., L. Cima, and P. Costa. 1988. Bioaccumulation of Hg in the mushroom Pleurotus ostreatus. Ecotoxicology and Environmental Safety Oct. 16: 85-89.

7) Canadian Cancer Society, 2010. Chemotherapy: A Guide for People with Cancer. Toronto, Canada. 52pp.

8) Canadian Cancer Society's Steering Committee on Cancer Statistics. Canadian Cancer Statistics 2014. Toronto, Ontario: Canadian Cancer Society; 2014. 132pp.

9) Colorectal Cancer Association of Canada, 2010. Screening and diagnosis: Pet and colorectal cancer. Available at http://www.colorectal-cancer.ca/en/screening/pet-cancer/. Accessed on 7th June 2013.

10) ConvaTec, 2009. Living with Confidence after Ostomy Surgery. Customer Relations Center. ConvaTec Inc. Canada. 43pp.

11) Copeland K., 1997. You Are Healed. Eagle Mountain International Church Inc./Kenneth Copeland Ministries Inc. Fort Worth, Texas. 33pp.

12) Copeland K. and Copeland G., 1992. From Faith To Faith: A Daily Guide To Victory. Eagle Mountain International Church Inc./Kenneth Copeland Ministries Inc. Fort Worth, Texas.

13) Dawn Soo, 2002. The potential of fungi used in traditional Chinese medicine: Shiitake (Lentinula edodes). Downloaded from the World of Fungi internet website: [http://www.world-of-ungi.org/Mostly Medical/ Dawn Soo/Dawn Soo SSM.html].

14) Dollinger, M., Rosenbaum, E., Tempero, M. and S. Mulvihill, 2002. Everyone's Guide to Cancer Therapy: How Cancer Is Diagnosed, Treated and Managed Day to Day. (4th Edition). Kansas City: Andrews McMeel Publishing. 1: pp. 3-16.

15) FAO/WHO, 1993. Joint FAO/WHO Food Standard Programme, Codex Alimentarius Commission, 24 th Session, 2-7 July, report on the 32 nd session of the Codex Committee on Food Additives and Contaminants ALINORM 01/12, 20-24 March 2000 in Beijing, People's Republic of China. Geneva, Switzerland.

16) FAO/WHO, 2001. Joint FAO/WHO Food Standard Programme, Codex Alimentarius Commission: Report on the 8th session of the Codex Committee on cereals, pulses and legumes in Washington, 1992. Geneva, Switzerland.

17) Ingram, S., 2002. The real nutritional value of fungi. Downloaded from internet site: [http://www.world-of-fungi.org/Mostly Medical/Stephanie Ingram/ NUTRITIONAL VALUE.htm].

18) International Agency for Research on Cancer/WHO (2013). Biannual Report 2012-2013. SC/52/2; SC/56/2. IARC, Lyon, France. 174pp.

19) Leslie, J.F., 2005. Diversity in toxigenic Fusarium species in Africa. Workshop on reducing impact of mycotoxins in tropical agriculture with emphasis on health and trade in Africa. 13-16 September 2005. Accra, Ghana.

20) Marasas, W.F.O., N.PJ. Kriek, M. Steyn, S.J. van Rensburg and DJ. van Scbalkwyk, 1977. Mycotoxicological

investigations on Zambian maize. Cosmetic Toxicology 16: 39-45.

21) Marks, J.W., 2012. What is cancer of the colon and rectum? National Cancer Institute at the National Institute of Health. Available at http://www.medicinenet.com/ colon cancer/article.htm. Accessed on 2013.

22) Miller, D. and W. Marasas, 2002. Ecology of Mycotoxins in Maize and Groundnuts. Supplement to LEISA magazine. Pages 23-24. ICRISAT.

23) National Cancer Institute, 2006. What You Need To Know About™ Cancer. Maryland, USA. 66pp.

24) National Cancer Institute-PDQ 2013. Colon Cancer Treatment: Patient Version available at http://www.ncbi.nlm.nih.gov/pubmedhealth/ PMH0032664/#CDR0000062954 93. Accessed on October 16, 2013.

25) National Cancer Institute: PDQ® [Cancer Information Summaries: Colon Cancer Treatment-Patient Version]. Bethesda, MD. National Cancer Institute. Last Update: September 20, 2013. Available at http://www.ncbi.nlm.nih. gov/pubmedhealth/PMH0032664/#CDR0000062954 93. Accessed March/04/2014.

26) National Cancer Institute: PDQ®, 2014. What is Cancer? Defining cancer. Last updated: March 7, 2014. Available at http://www.cancer.gov/cancertopics/cancerlibrary/what-is-cancer. Accessed February 10, 2015.

27) Osteen D., 2003. Healed Of cancer. A Lakewood Church Publication. Houston, Texas. 81pp.

28) Ottawa Hospital Cancer Center, 2010. Chemotherapy Home Infusion Pump Program (CHIPP): Questions and Answers for Patients, Families and Friends. Ottawa Hospital. Ottawa, Canada. 20pp.

29) Overstory, 2004. The role of mushrooms in nature. The Overstory No. 84. The Overstory Agroforetry eJournal. [www.overstory.org].

30) Pagels D. (ed.), 2010. Faith Will See You Through. Blue Mountain Arts, Inc. Boulder, Colorado. USA.

31) Parkin, D.M., J. Ferlay, M. Hamdi-Chérif, F. Sites, J.O. Thomas, H. Wabinga and S.L. Whelan, 2003. Cancer in Africa: Epidemiology and Prevention. International Agency for Research on Cancer – World Health Organization. Scientific Publications No. 153. IARCPressLyon. Lyon, France. 414pp.

32) Sikombwa, N. and G.D. Piearce, 1985. Vanderbylia ungulata and its medicinal use in Zambia. Bulletin of the British Mycological Society 19: 124-125.

33) Spangler, A., 2004. Praying the Names of God: A Daily Guide. Zondervan Co. Grand Rapids. Michigan, USA. 348pp.

34) Stijve, T. 1992. Certain mushrooms do accumulate heavy metals. Mushroom, The Journal of Wild Mushrooming 38: 9-14.

35) Stijve, T. and R. Roschnik. 1974. Mercury and methyl mercury content of different species of Fungi. Trav. Chim. Alimen. Hyg. 65:209-220.

36) The Ottawa Hospital, 2010. Patient Information on Bowel Resection: Minimal Invasive Surgery (MIS) and Open Surgery. Ottawa, Canada. 26pp.

37) The Ottawa Hospital, 2012. Guide: Pain Management after Surgery. Ottawa, Canada. 24pp.

38) West, R.M., 2007. How To Study The Bible. Barbour Publishing Inc. Uhrichsville, Ohio. USA. 95pp.

39) Williams, J.H., T. D. Phillips, P.E. Jolly, J.K. Stiles, C.M. Jolly and D. Aggarwal, 2004. Human aflatoxicosis in developing countries: A review of toxicology, exposure, potential health consequences, and interventions. Am. J. Clin. Nutr. 80:1106-1122.

40) World Health Organization (WHO), 2007. The World Health Organization's Fight Against Cancer: Strategies that Prevent, Cure and Care. Geneva, Switzerland. 24pp.

41) WHO, 2009. Exposure of children to chemical hazards in food. Fact sheet 4.4, Code: RPG4 Food Ex1. European Environment and Health Information System (ENHIS). Available at http://www.euro.who.int/ENHIS.

42) WHO, 2013. Global Health Observatory (GHO), Cancer mortality and morbidity. Cancer. Reviewed Fact sheet N°297, 2013. (http://www.who.int/mediacentre/factsheets/fs297/en/index.html). Accessed on 2013.

Other reading resources

1) American Institute for Cancer Research, 2013. AICR's foods that fight cancer. Available at http://www.aicr.org/foods-that-fight-cancer/. Accessed on 2013.

2) Bayshore Home Health Care. Available at http://www.bayshore.ca. Accessed on 2013.

3) Carefor Health and Community Services. Available at http://www.carefor.ca. Accessed on 2013.

4) Colorectal Cancer Association of Canada, 2013. Canadian cancer patients need better access to latest drugs, therapy: Report. Available at http://www.colorectal-cancer.ca. Accessed on 2013.

5) Community Care Access Centre. Available at at http://www.ccac-ont.ca. Accessed on 2013.

6) Ottawa Regional Cancer Foundation. Available at http://www.ottawacancer.ca. Accessed on 2013.

7) WHO, 2013. Cancer: Early detection of cancer. Available at http://www.who.int/cancer/detection/en/. Accessed on 2013.

INDEX